PRAISE

EAT TO BEAT DEPRES

T0268122

"Dr. Ramsey has been a pioneer of the n̲_____
and of promoting the use of nutrition in mental health. His new book really explains why that is with ample evidence, beautiful illustrations, actionable steps, and stellar recipes. Essential reading for anyone seeking to build mental health and wellness."

—Mark Hyman, MD, Pritzker Foundation chair in functional
medicine, Cleveland Clinic Lerner College of Medicine,
and twelve-time New York Times bestselling author

"In a world where depression and anxiety are increasingly common and painfully corrosive to our lives, Dr. Ramsey provides a beautiful and clear road map to help us move from lonely suffering to rich, meaningful living through simple dietary shifts. This book distills powerful advice into bite-size recommendations, and Dr. Ramsey does a wonderful job of connecting our choices to our experiences so that we know not only what to do but why. I will be sharing this book with many, many people."

—Dallas Hartwig, cocreator of Whole30 and author of
The 4 Season Solution

"Dr. Ramsey has been leading the world of mental health to food and nutrition. I know the power of food to improve brain health. This is a must-have book for people struggling with depression or anxiety."

—Terry Wahls, MD, clinical professor of medicine at the
University of Iowa Carver College of Medicine and
author of The Wahls Protocol

"*Eat to Beat Depression and Anxiety* reminds us all that prevention is the best medicine. Ramsey thoughtfully weaves together elements of nutrition, psychiatry, and public health to provide practical lifestyle recommendations rooted in scientific evidence. As our country continues to face an unprecedented mental health crisis, we must all think carefully about the ways in which we nourish ourselves."

—Former US Rep. Patrick J. Kennedy, cofounder of Psych Hub

"Dr. Ramsey is a psychiatrist, author, farmer, *and* a leading proponent that food is medicine! In *Eat to Beat Depression and Anxiety*, Drew shares his deep personal insights on both nutrition and psychiatry, unveiling a truth I wholeheartedly endorse: What we eat impacts our mental health."

—Lisa Mosconi, PhD, director of the Weill Cornell Women's Brain
Initiative and author of New York Times bestselling The XX Brain

"Dr. Ramsey is one of the few brave voices in the medical community who is experienced, courageous, and confident enough to talk openly about food and its significance on mental health. What you choose to put on your plate is one of the most important health interventions and Dr. Drew has written a fantastic resource for patients and colleagues alike, to take control of their health using their fork. I'm personally inspired by Drew's work and the immense effort he brings to all of his books and projects."

—Dr. Rupy Aujla, founder and author of *The Doctor's Kitchen*

"Dr. Drew Ramsey was one of my earliest inspirations and supporters in my work in culinary medicine. He has a unique skill of translating the science of nutritional psychiatry in approachable, user-friendly, fun and delicious ways. I am so excited to use *Eat to Beat Nutrition and Anxiety* in my clinical practice to help my patients eat well, and feel better."

—Linda Shiue, MD, chef, director of Culinary Medicine,
Author of *Spicebox Kitchen*

"*Eat to Beat Depression and Anxiety* provides an engaging, personable, and evidence-based approach about how making the right food choices can improve your mood and allow you to feel happier. This book is a must-have for anyone who cares about food and is interested in feeling good."

—Gregory Scott Brown, MD, psychiatrist and author

"Dr. Drew Ramsey is a wonderful psychiatrist committed to innovation in mental health care and the inclusion of food and nutrition. He is one of the few psychiatrists I'd like to cook me dinner and my only colleague who owns a tractor! His latest book teaches us to nourish our brains to improve mood and decrease anxiety. This is Ramsey at his best, weaving brain health, food, and his passion for mental wellness."

—Lloyd I. Sederer, MD, adjunct professor, Columbia University
School of Public Health, and director of Columbia Psychiatry Media

"My father was a psychiatrist and my mother was a cookbook author. *Eat to Beat Depression and Anxiety* marries the two professions into a conversation that we never had at the dinner table growing up—the connection between food and mood. Dr. Ramsey's book is a must-read and will shift your relationship with food to be more mindful with a perspective on culinary medicine."

—Marjorie Morrison, LMFT, LPC, CEO and cofounder, Psych Hub

ALSO BY DREW RAMSEY

....

Eat Complete

Fifty Shades of Kale

The Happiness Diet

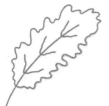

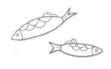
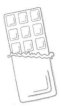

EAT TO BEAT DEPRESSION AND ANXIETY

Nourish Your Way to Better Mental Health in Six Weeks

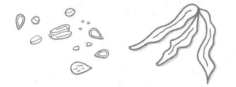

DREW RAMSEY, MD

HARPER

NEW YORK · LONDON · TORONTO · SYDNEY

To my colleagues working in mental health.
Keep up the good fight.

HARPER

A hardcover edition of this book was published in 2021 by Harper, and imprint of HarperCollins Publishers.

HarperCollins books may be purchased for educational, business, or sales promotional use. For information, please email the Special Markets Department at SPsales@harpercollins.com.

FIRST HARPER PAPERBACK EDITION PUBLISHED 2025.

Illustrations by Katrin Wietek

Library of Congress Cataloging-in-Publication Data has been applied for.

ISBN 978-0-06-303172-2 (pbk.)

24 25 26 27 28 LBC 5 4 3 2 1

CONTENTS

Introduction. vii

Part I Eating for Optimal Mental Health

Chapter 1 THE NEW SCIENCE OF EATING FOR MENTAL HEALTH . . . 3

Chapter 2 TWELVE NUTRIENTS FOR A BETTER BRAIN 19

Chapter 3 HOW TO GROW NEW BRAIN CELLS 55

Chapter 4 OPTIMIZE YOUR GUT FOR MENTAL HEALTH 77

Chapter 5 THE BEST FOODS TO BEAT DEPRESSION
AND ANXIETY. 95

Part II Get Started: Your Path to Healing

Chapter 6 CHALLENGES FACING THE MODERN EATER 117

Chapter 7 EATER, HEAL THYSELF 139

Chapter 8 THE KITCHEN. 153

Chapter 9 THE SIX-WEEK PLAN AND RECIPES 173

Acknowledgments 237

Resources 241

Notes 247

Index 251

INTRODUCTION

Psychiatric medicine and mental healthcare have a serious problem.

Experts around the globe—from the World Health Organization to the Pew Research Center—all agree: we are in the midst of a mental health epidemic. Diagnoses of depression and anxiety disorders have snowballed over the past decade, now occurring more frequently in teens and young children. The number of suicides across the United States has skyrocketed during this time as well to a level beyond tragic. Anyone reading the headlines is aware that substance abuse issues are at an all-time high, too. Approximately one in four individuals will be diagnosed with a mental health condition, like depression or anxiety, over the course of their life. Chances are, you or someone close to you has struggled with a mental health issue at some point.

In some ways, these statistics are not surprising. Our health is being challenged in ways we simply could not have anticipated even just a few years ago. Today, as a society, we are overworked, overstressed, and overstimulated by the demands of daily life. We eat too much, sleep too little, remain too sedentary, and discount what our bodies need to truly thrive. The modern Western lifestyle has wreaked havoc on our physical health, leading to increased incidence of medical conditions like diabetes, cancer, and heart disease. This lifestyle has greatly affected our mental health, too. More and more, people go about their days with depleted energy stores, feelings of hopelessness, and an overwhelming sense of worry. We seem to be at the mercy of our devices and smartphones, spending far too much time distracted by strangers instead of making strong connections with those closest to us. Over time, all these things add up, leading to mental health crises—and, perhaps, a clinical diagnosis.

Given this ongoing battle to preserve America's mental health, patients, families, and doctors need all the tools they can get to win this fight. Over the past few decades, the field of psychiatry has gained remarkable insights into the biological factors that may underlie changes in mood and anxiety levels. Yet emerging scientific studies are now showing us that one of the most powerful—and underutilized—tools to help us combat depression and anxiety can be found at the end of your fork.

THE MISSING PIECE OF THE PUZZLE

Today I'm known as a nutritional psychiatrist. But I didn't always know that food played such a vital role in brain health.

As a practicing psychiatrist who specializes in mood and anxiety disorders, my job is to review and assess a patient's complete medical history to get to the bottom of any mental health issue. My training helps me understand that physical and mental health are intrinsically linked—for example, often a bodily issue like a thyroid problem can have great impact on a person's mood or anxiety levels. During an initial workup, psychiatrists will ask patients a lot of questions, some of which they may not expect to be asked, to gather the data needed to understand what may be at the root of a person's low mood or increased feelings of anxiety. When I was just starting out in my career, I learned a lot about how to ask questions about a person's medical history, family background, and what might be happening at work and at home.

But I'd never been taught to ask my patients what they were eating.

This struck me, even then, as a bit odd. That's likely because of my background. In the late seventies, when I was five years old, my parents moved our family from Long Island, New York, to a homestead in Crawford County, Indiana. There, they started caring for 123 acres of pasture farmland, planting, tending, and harvesting a variety of fruit, vegetables, greens, beans, and herbs. Today, I live on that same farm with my wife, children, and parents, commuting each week to my clinic in New York City. I spend my weekends battling the dense clay soil, weather, and bugs—and marveling, with my children, at the miracle of seeds sprouting into nourishing food. I may not have been fully conscious of it at the time, but even as a child, I seemed to understand that eating fresh, whole foods just made me feel better—in body, mind, and spirit.

Years later, while a medical student at Indiana University, what I learned about nutrition can most succinctly be summed up as "meat and dairy are bad, vegetables are good." It's probably not so different from what you've read over the years about what constitutes a healthy diet. And so, wanting to be happier and healthier, I decided to adopt a low-fat vegetarian diet. In fact, I didn't eat meat, including fish and seafood, for nearly twelve years.

While the data is clear that eating mainly plant-based foods plays an important role in overall health, I was so focused on maintaining a diet without steak or salmon that I didn't stop to consider whether my body—and my brain—were getting the nutrients they needed to truly thrive. My go-to foods included veggie burgers, mac and cheese, and a lot of pizza. It wasn't until new research started to link levels of omega-3 fatty acids, a type of polyunsaturated fatty acids commonly found in seafood, to brain health that I started to wonder if maybe my diet wasn't as healthy as I'd thought.

I began to wonder: are there foods that can better help promote brain and mental health? And, if so, why aren't we talking about those foods, and how they affect mood and anxiety?

A NEW PRESCRIPTION—FOR FOOD

Traditionally, treatment protocols for depression and anxiety have focused on talk therapy and medication. These two tools, working alone or in tandem, work well for many people, when they're available. Unfortunately, for others, these popular interventions do not bring as much relief as hoped—or if they do, they come with a host of unpleasant side effects, including weight gain, drowsiness, sexual problems, and constipation. This can demoralize patients who are already struggling to just feel even a little bit better.

As a physician, who swore an oath to "do no harm," it's important to me to explore all the available options to help my patients feel better. And, as part of that, I also want to make sure anything I prescribe isn't just replacing one health issue with another. While antidepressant and antipsychotic medications have changed the face of psychiatry, and have been lifesavers for many patients, they cannot and should not be the only tools at a psychiatrist's disposal to treat patients. Any safe, effective options we can add to our arsenal to help prevent, manage, or remit mental health conditions are more than welcome.

Healthy eating is one such tool. Yet good, nourishing foods that provide key nutrients setting the foundation for optimal brain function have been all but overlooked in the mental health arena. At this point, it's hard to understand why. The science is clear. We've known for over a decade that your dietary pattern, or the amount and variety of foods you habitually consume, is linked to brain function, and, by extension, your risk of developing a condition like depression or anxiety. Good mental health, just like physical health, depends on proper nutrition. If you are running low on a few key vitamins or minerals, you are more likely to experience issues with mood or excessive worrying. So why not focus on ways to increase those vital nutrients?

When I did finally start talking to my patients about what they ate, the results were startling, to say the least. Not only were the vast majority of them not eating the healthy nutrients that we now know are vital to maintaining a thriving body and brain, but they were also actively consuming foods that we know to be detrimental to their health. It became clear to me that here was a place where we, as clinicians, could better support our patients as they underwent treatment. And, in the process, empower them to make positive changes on their own to help improve their own mental health.

Despite the fact that a flood of studies has now been published demonstrating that good, nutrient-dense food really is a form of medicine, both in terms of physical and mental health, many of my colleagues are still approaching depression and anxiety in the same old ways. That needs to change. Luckily, you don't need to rely on a mental health practitioner to make the kind of dietary changes needed to improve your mental health. You can learn how to best nourish your brain—and yourself—and start eating to beat depression and anxiety.

THIS BOOK IS FOR EATERS

There's a reason why you picked up this book. Maybe you or a loved one have been diagnosed with depression or anxiety. Perhaps you're experiencing feelings of decreased motivation—or you find yourself worrying more than you'd like. Over the past decade, we now understand both depression and anxiety can start from a lot of different places. But what we've seen in my clinic is that nutrition can play a pivotal role in helping to manage the symptoms of these two common clinical disorders in conjunction with medication, psychotherapy, or other interventions. That said, you don't have to wait to have a clinical diagnosis in order to reap the benefits of a brain-healthy diet. If you're experiencing fatigue, brain fog, mood swings, or unrelenting worries, introducing more high-quality food into your diet, with the right nutrients to help your brain work its best, can help. Everyone with a brain should know how to feed it for optimal functioning. I hope this book will help you do just that.

Whether you're looking to increase your energy levels or just want to do a better job of nourishing your family, understanding why food is such an integral part of mental health is the first step in the journey of self-nourishment. You've probably heard a lot of confusing information about diet and its impact on health over the years. Every few months, there seems to be a new fad diet that everyone is talking about. These plans often tell you there is a single, "right" way to eat. They might tell you *never* to prepare food this way—and, while you're at it, eliminate this food from your diet altogether. They may say that you need to add another food to every single meal without fail. Or eat certain foods only in specific combinations. These diets tend to come with complicated meal plans that you are expected to follow to the letter. They may even have a sideline of supplements to sell you.

Then, like clockwork, some other popular diet will come out a few months later, contradicting all you thought was good and healthy. The only thing this diet will have in common with the last one is the message that you are eating all wrong. With so much inconsistent information regarding food and health, is it any wonder that so many of us are suffering from some form of nutritional fatigue? As you try to make sense of so many conflicting studies and diet plans, it's hard to know what is truly evidence-based and scientifically sound—and what can really help you as you strive for optimal brain health.

Unfortunately, much of the guidance you get from others about the best way to treat depression and anxiety may be just as confusing. If you or someone you love has clinical depression or anxiety, it's likely you've already received your fair share of advice about how to manage it. Maybe someone has told you to be more positive—or to just calm down and not worry so much! You may have been asked if you've tried yoga or Transcendental Meditation. Someone may have suggested you look into adult coloring books or essential oils. A few may have even ventured to recommend a particular antidepressant medication to you. After all, it worked wonders for someone they know.

That's why I want to say up front that this is not a diet book, nor is it a book that suggests that food is a panacea for mental health conditions. Rather, this is a book for eaters, pure and simple. Being a psychiatrist interested in food sometimes makes people worried that I'm judging what they eat. I tell my patients all the time that I'm not in the judgment business. No one is looking to blame you or shame you for the way you eat. My work with patients has taught me to respect that each of you has unique tastes and values about food that are as individual as your experiences with depression and anxiety. I understand that it can be difficult to change ingrained habits regarding what and how you eat, especially when you aren't feeling your best. That's why there is no "must do" advice in the following pages.

TAKING THE FIRST STEPS

I'll be straight with you. There is no one right way to implement what you learn here, no stringent protocol or unyielding meal plans. I won't even tell you that you must eat certain foods, but instead I will highlight different food categories, based on the newest science, that contain the vital nutrients your brain needs to prevent and treat depression and anxiety.

What you'll find in the following chapters is evidence-based knowledge about how food can affect your brain health. And, with that, I hope you'll gain the confidence and know-how to make a few small changes or substitutions that work for you, your family, and your lifestyle. Believe it or not, it's the small changes that can have big effects when it comes to your mood and anxiety levels. Eating to beat depression and anxiety is about understanding the connections between the foods you eat and your brain, learning how to

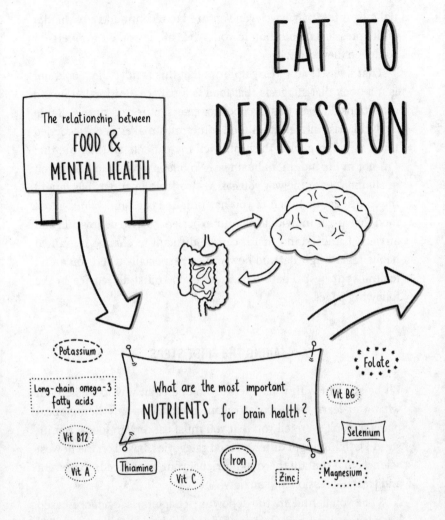

EAT TO DEPRESSION

The relationship between FOOD & MENTAL HEALTH

Potassium

Long-chain omega-3 fatty acids

Vit B12

Vit A   Thiamine   Vit C   Iron   Zinc   Magnesium

What are the most important NUTRIENTS for brain health?

Folate

Vit B6

Selenium

eat for more brain-nutrient density, and finding your own way to becoming a master of self-nourishment.

To help get you started, I've laid out a six-week plan within these pages intended to deepen your connection to your food. I'll start by asking you to prioritize your brain health, as your brain is the most important organ in your body—and, as such, the one that

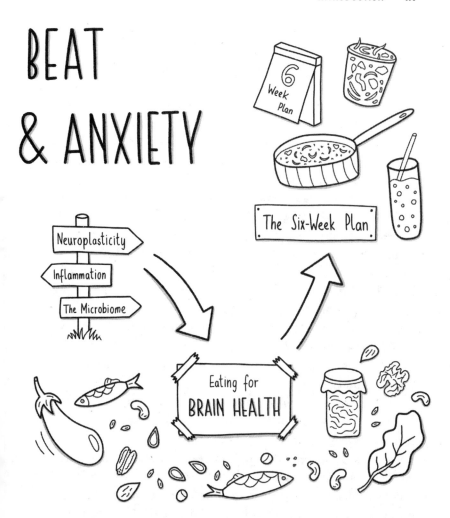

should most influence your food choices. For a lot of people, eating for brain health will require a few changes to how you think about food, dismissing the "good" and "bad" labels that have been attached to certain food categories over the years. It may also entail addressing challenges you may have about different foods—and, at the very least, trying some foods that you might have dismissed before. Case in point, my wife recently and quite unexpectedly fell in love with fish roe after trying them for the first time. That was a pretty big surprise. But, ultimately, what you eat is entirely up to you.

This book is about helping you tap into the most powerful act of self-care known to humankind: feeding yourself. While so many headlines referencing Nutritional Psychiatry studies highlight individual nutrients or foods, this isn't about just adding more kale or a zinc supplement to your diet. Certainly, it's compelling to learn that the regular consumption of leafy greens is strongly correlated with a reduction in inflammation, an immune process that has been linked to depression, but this is also about looking more deeply into yourself and your food choices and what steps you can take to consume the foods that support and nurture your brain. Conditions like depression and anxiety can alter the way we feel and think about ourselves and our environment—so it's not surprising they also tend to change the way we eat. But using food, in addition to other tools, to equip and empower us as we look for relief from depression and anxiety symptoms can play a significant role in recovery.

In an era of sensational, and often confusing, nutritional advice, I want to provide you with a balanced and informed view on nutrition and how it affects brain health. From the pros and cons of eating meat to the best brain-healthy seafood choices, my ultimate goal is to provide you with the confidence to know, with each and every bite, that you're eating to improve your mental health. You're eating to give your brain the nutrients it needs to function at its best. You're eating to beat depression and anxiety.

PART I

Eating for Optimal
Mental Health

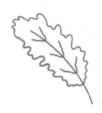

THE NEW SCIENCE OF EATING FOR MENTAL HEALTH

What Should Pete and Susan Eat?

Over the past decade, the Food Is Medicine movement has gained tremendous momentum. Primary care physicians, cardiologists, and oncologists now understand that what you put into your mouth at each meal strongly influences your overall health. In fact, you were likely asked some general questions about your diet at your last annual physical—or were at least given a handout about a heart-healthy diet before you went home. Yet despite those strides forward in other fields of medicine, mental health practitioners, for the most part, are not following suit. We know that what's good for the body is good for the brain—but discussions about food remain the exception, not the rule, in the assessment and treatment of common conditions like depression and anxiety.

The emerging field of Nutritional Psychiatry is a new and growing movement focused on the use of nutrition to optimize brain health and, in doing so, help prevent and treat mental health concerns. A flood of new and exciting scientific studies is now demonstrating that, as with physical health, our food choices affect our mental well-being. They show the impact of specific nutrients, including omega-3 fats, zinc, and different plant-based molecules, on brain health. They reveal the complex relationship between inflammation and brain function. They explain how the microbiome—the trillions of bacteria that live within each of our guts—influences mood, cognition, and an individual's overall risk of mental illness. It's important to note that such studies now also include several randomized clinical trials illustrating that targeted changes to a person's diet, increasing the vital nutrients that promote brain health, can help improve mood and lessen feelings of anxiety.

Put it all together and we know the foods we pick to feed and nourish ourselves directly influence our risk of developing depression and anxiety—and those same foods can also assist in keeping common symptoms associated with these conditions in check. Given that eating is the most fundamental act of self-care—and is an area where we each can be empowered to enhance our own mental health—these new findings in Nutritional Psychiatry truly are a game changer.

Take Pete, a young man in his twenties who came to me for treatment a few years ago. Some might say Pete was suffering from a "failure to launch." After finishing college, he was unable to find a job and had to move back in with his parents. He felt like his friends had all moved on with their lives and found some version of success, but he was "stuck in place." He had a history of depression, which started when he was a teenager, and had been faithfully taking an antidepressant medication for years. When he walked into my office, Pete explained to me that he didn't feel like the meds were working as well, if at all, anymore. His parents, naturally, were quite worried.

During our first meeting, Pete told me he feels "down and pretty dark" most of the time. He felt like he was disappointing his parents. He felt like he was disappointing himself. And he wasn't sure how to get back to feeling more, as he put it, "normal."

"I notice I don't look up anymore," Pete said. "It's weird. I'm always looking down."

As we talked more, I learned that Pete rarely left his bedroom, let alone the house. He wasn't connecting with friends or family as well as he used to—and no longer had the energy to engage in activities that he used to enjoy, like soccer or trivia nights. His sleep patterns also were an issue. He would stay up until the wee hours playing video games, and then wake up around 1 or 2 p.m. the next day.

When I asked him to describe his eating habits to me, it became clear he was subsisting on what you might call the twelve-year-old boy diet. Upon waking each afternoon, he said, he'd just eat whatever he found in his parents' fridge. Lots of processed foods. Lots of sugar. Lots of carbohydrates. Lots of easy, microwavable meals with lots of salt, food dyes, and trans fats—and, of course, very little nutritional value. As he told me about his dietary pattern, it became clear that food was an area where we could make some small improvements, likely to great effect. I prescribed a few simple food swaps, like replacing his favorite Mexican takeout with some fish tacos and adding a handful of greens to his "morning" smoothie, to help Pete, and Pete's brain, get the nutrients they so desperately needed. I asked Pete to go to the grocery store with his mom and to cook a bit more, maybe swap chips and cookies for nuts. At first, Pete was skeptical, but, within a few sessions, he started to make steady progress forward.

Several months later, he told me, "I just know if I don't eat right, I don't feel right." Today, Pete makes sure his diet contains enough seafood, leafy greens, and rainbow vegetables to help bolster his mood. Within a few months, we were able to significantly decrease the dosage of his medication.

It may seem like making a few tweaks to Pete's diet as an intervention for depression is too good to be true, but think of it this way: the brain is an expensive machine to run. Despite only weighing about three pounds, the human brain consumes about 20 percent of the calories you eat each day. Its optimal functioning depends upon a dozen key nutrients—the vitamins, minerals, fats, and proteins that provide the brain with the building blocks and supporting molecules required to back its cells, neurotransmitters, and insulating white matter. That's why assessing nutrition and food choices should be an integral part of the paradigm for treating and preventing mental health disorders—and why doing this worked so well for Pete, in addition to his medication and talk therapy sessions.

Another patient, Susan, might seem like your stereotypical high-strung middle-aged mom. In her late thirties, Susan couldn't help but carry the weight of the world on her shoulders. She incessantly worried about her work, marriage, three kids, and ill eighty-two-year-old mother. She'd watch the news each night and feel her heart rate elevating as the latest political fight unfolded on her favorite cable news show. Often, when her husband tried to strike up a conversation with her over dinner, she had trouble concentrating on what he was saying. Instead of actively listening, she was too busy fretting over something that happened earlier in the day, replaying it over and over again in her head.

I probably don't have to add that Susan was also having trouble getting to bed and staying asleep each night. Often, she would drink a couple glasses of wine before bed to help calm down and, as she puts it, "feel more evened out." But then, she said, she would worry that she was becoming too dependent on the alcohol to help her relax. "I just lie there and think about all the things I didn't get done during the day," she told me. "And then I worry about what's going on with the kids, and my mom, and the world at large. It's really quite overwhelming."

Susan came to me to help with strategies to better manage her anxiety. After doing a full medical workup, we started talking about what she eats in an average week. Susan takes great pride in eating healthy, which to her meant low-calorie and low-fat—but trying to plan meals with her and her family's busy schedule often would become just another thing for her to become anxious about.

"It seems like I'm always running somewhere," she said. "There's more takeout than I'd like for all of us but there never seems to be time for anything else."

As Susan shared what her meals looked like over a week, I noticed she did try to make what she believed to be healthy food choices, avoiding fried foods and sugary drinks. But she also rarely ate eggs, nuts, or seafood. She generally didn't bother with breakfast. Her go-to meal was a basic iceberg lettuce salad with grilled chicken, a couple of cucumber slices, and a simple canola oil vinaigrette. Like with Pete, it was easy for me to see some places where she could make a few key changes, like replacing canola oil with olive oil and adding more nutrient-dense leafy greens to her salads. I also suggested that she start having eggs several mornings a week for breakfast, ensuring she was starting her day with essential nutrients like protein, B vitamins, and choline.

We also talked about ways she could prep meals in advance, so there would always be healthy options available to her and her family even during her busiest weeks. Within a few months, the combination of those changes and talk therapy helped Susan find a little more confidence and a lot more calm in her life, allowing her to better harness the different strategies she'd learned to keep her anxiety levels in check.

If Pete or Susan had seen another psychiatrist, they likely would never have been asked what they were eating. Yet, in both cases, asking about their dietary patterns uncovered areas where Pete and Susan could empower themselves to make improvements in their brain health—and, by extension, their mental health. This is not to say that food was the only factor in their recoveries. Overcoming depression and anxiety often require other tools, like our go-to interventions of medication and psychotherapy. But, for many people, eating a diet filled with foods that support brain health makes those more traditional treatments work all the better.

These are only two examples where applying the principles of Nutritional Psychiatry helped my patients better manage their conditions. If you looked at the case files in my clinic, you'd see dozens and dozens more. As the evidence base rapidly grows for the relationship between food choices and mood and anxiety disorders, it's imperative that doctors ask their patients probing questions about what they eat—and that you, as someone who may be struggling with your mood or anxiety levels, know which foods can best nourish your brain. After all, if food is medicine, it's also medicine for the brain.

DEFINING DEPRESSION AND ANXIETY

Terms like "depression" and "anxiety" are used in a variety of ways in everyday conversations. You hear them talked about in books, movies, and your favorite television shows. With both terms used so widely, it's not surprising that they often mean different things to different people. That said, it's important to note that both depression and anxiety are clinical mental health disorders. The fifth edition of the *Diagnostic and Statistical Manual of Mental Disorders* (DSM-5), the reference book used by healthcare professionals to help them diagnose mental health conditions, provides a list of symptoms that we look to when we assess our patients and determine if they have one of these brain illnesses. But as you start to think about ways you might eat to beat depression or anxiety, it's important to understand what these terms really mean.

We tend to talk about depression as the experience of consistently feeling sad or hopeless. In psychiatry and medicine, doctors try to differentiate whether those feelings are due to some kind of situation happening in your life, like a traumatic breakup, the death of a family member, or some sort of biological issue, that would lead to a diagnosis of a major depressive episode. The DSM-5 defines depression as a person having multiple symptoms, which may include a depressed mood, loss of energy, diminished ability to concentrate, changes in appetite, and decreased interest or pleasure in normally enjoyable activities, for more than a two-week period. It also states that depression is disruptive, meaning that a person's decreased mood is interfering with their ability to comfortably live their lives. A person with depression may have a lot of trouble getting out of bed in the morning, finishing basic tasks, or connecting with friends and family. One of my patients once described depression to me as what happens when life loses its color—and I think that's a very illuminating description.

Anxiety, on the other hand, is often characterized as a sort of extreme bout of worry. That description is not too far off the mark, but people experience anxiety to varying degrees. The DSM-5 defines generalized anxiety disorder, the most common anxiety disorder, as "excessive anxiety or worry," with symptoms that may include feeling "keyed up," irritability, fatigue, and sleep troubles. To be diagnosed with anxiety, you would be experiencing some of those symptoms more days than not over a six-month period. Like with depression, psychiatrists try to differentiate a situational anxiety, perhaps due to a chaotic time at work or a challenging life transition, to a cause that may be rooted in neurobiology.

Let me further explain: the human brain has evolved to have an essential "alarm system" that helps us survive. Think about the most fundamental survival reaction, the so-called fight-or-flight response. In response to a stressful situation, the brain will ramp up stress hormones, including one called cortisol, to help better prepare you to deal with the situation at hand. So, a little anxiety can be a good thing. It can help us up our cognitive game, preparing us to perform well before a big test, a sporting event, or just a drive home on an icy road at night. But when that alarm system steadily misfires, flooding the brain with stress hormones in situations that don't require that sort of vigilant response, clinical anxiety issues sometimes start to take root. That's when you'll see the worry really start to ramp up and, with it, sleep problems, gastrointestinal issues, and even, sometimes, physical pain. Like depression, anxiety really becomes a problem when it starts to intrude upon your day-to-day life, interfering with your work and your relationships.

Treating these conditions isn't as easy as you might think. Despite the development of many effective antidepressant and anti-anxiety medications, not everyone responds to them in the same way. More than ten years ago, the National Institute of Mental Health (NIMH) published a landmark study, the Sequenced Treatment Alternatives to Relieve Depression (STAR*D). This study looked at the efficacy of several common antidepressant treatments like selective serotonin reuptake inhibitors (SSRIs) such as Prozac and Zoloft and cognitive behavioral therapy (CBT). The study found a whopping two-thirds of participants didn't find relief after being prescribed a single antidepressant medication. Most had to try several different medications before they saw a significant drop in their symptoms—but their doctors had to go through a mostly trial-and-error process to get there. And, even after all that, 62 percent of patients either dropped out of the study or didn't feel better with treatment.

We see a similar pattern in medications to treat anxiety disorders.[1] Medications, too often, offer "incomplete" remission from symptoms. As a practitioner who works hard to help my patients feel better, that's alarming. While we know that psychiatric medications help millions of people, they aren't the be-all and end-all in treatment.

These studies, taken together, show us that we need to do more than write a prescription for a medicine to help people striving to beat depression and anxiety. We need to take a more complementary approach, including many forms of psychotherapy—better known as talk therapy—as well as careful inventory of lifestyle factors, like diet and exercise, to help design a more thorough approach to symptom management.

A note about anxiety: As you continue on with the following chapters, you may notice many of the studies described within these pages look at how different nutrients or food interventions affect depression—and only depression. If you picked up this book because of concerns about anxiety, I can understand that may be frustrating. Generalized anxiety disorder is the most commonly diagnosed mental health disorder in the United States. As a mental health practitioner, I, too, am dismayed that the link between food and anxiety by itself hasn't been more thoroughly investigated. Luckily, that is changing. But, that said, I would add that depression and anxiety often travel hand in hand. Many people are diagnosed with both conditions. They share some of the same symptoms. And when you look closely at the factors that can both cause and exacerbate these two mental health conditions, the overlaps are hard to miss. Those who work in the Nutritional Psychiatry field, like me, have learned firsthand that the kind of dietary changes that can prevent or better manage depression can do the same for anxiety disorders. And as you read on, and learn more about how inflammation and the microbiome affect the brain, I hope you'll better understand why that is.

THE TOP NUTRIENTS TO BEAT DEPRESSION AND ANXIETY

Research is telling us so much about depression and anxiety. Unfortunately, it often takes fifteen years or more for the latest scientific evidence to be integrated into clinical practice. No one should have to wait that long.

When I was in medical school, most clinicians agreed that, once you grew into adulthood, your brain was done growing. While the rest of the cells in the body would continue to reproduce throughout your life, you only got one set of brain cells—about a hundred billion or so—and, with luck, you'd manage not to kill too many off as you aged. Now, scientists have shown us that the brain, like the rest of the body, continues to change and grow well into our golden years. Its ability to continue to make new connections between cells is referred to as neuroplasticity. We are going to talk about neuroplasticity a lot more in Chapter 3. But for now, what's important to know is that neuroplasticity is one reason why consuming brain-healthy nutrients is so important to brain health. Those vitamins and minerals can provide the brain with the fuel it needs to promote healthy, dynamic growth.

A second reason why dietary patterns are so essential to brain health is that the foods we eat greatly influence bodily inflammation. The latest studies demonstrate that persistent, chronic inflammation—our immune system's protective response that helps to fight off injury or infection—can lead to depression and anxiety issues. A significant number of people who've been diagnosed with depression or anxiety show elevated levels of inflammatory proteins—and those molecules may be behind symptoms like anhedonia, or the inability to feel pleasure, and sleep issues.[2] Seasonal affective disorder (SAD), a type of depression that tends to hit in the late fall and early winter months, has also been linked to a higher level of inflammatory markers in the body.[3] There is a clear and strong link between inflammation and mood. Luckily, one of the most powerful tools available to combat this excess inflammation is food. By eating foods with anti-inflammatory properties, you can help reduce inflammation in the brain and, consequently, lower your risk of mental illness.

Other work is also showing the role of the microbiome, or the diverse population of bacteria and microbes that live within the human gut, to brain health. You might think those bacteria are there simply to help us digest and then take all that good energy from our food. We now understand that the brain and gut are in almost constant communication, and the so-called good bugs in the microbiome influence how our brain functions. Again, a nutrient-rich diet that contains probiotics from fermented foods can help promote the growth of those good bugs—and prevent depression and anxiety in the process.

Today, most doctors recommend that their patients eat a more Mediterranean-style diet. Eat like the Greeks and Italians do! It sounds easy enough. And, certainly, the Mediterranean diet has gotten a lot of attention over the past few years, especially as a means of reducing cholesterol and promoting heart health. Over time, science has shown us what's good for the heart is also good for the brain. We now understand the Mediterranean diet's focus on fruits, vegetables, fish, whole grains, and healthy fats provides the essential nutrients that support mental health by promoting neuroplasticity, fighting inflammation, and supporting all those good bugs living in your microbiome.

Yet, despite the success of the Mediterranean diet, I want to be able to give you more actionable advice on what kinds of foods can help manage conditions like depression and anxiety. In early 2016, my psychiatrist colleague Laura LaChance, MD, and I undertook a project to identify the nutrients that would offer patients suffering from depressive disorders the most bang for their buck, so to speak, in terms of reducing their depressive symptoms.

After reviewing all the published scientific research, Dr. LaChance and I created the Antidepressant Food Scale (AFS), highlighting the foods that contain the highest concentration of brain-boosting nutrients that can help fight depression. Our analysis identified twelve crucial nutrients that are involved with either the development or the treatment of depression—and we further noted the top plant and animal foods that contain those nutrients.

We'll go more in-depth in the next chapter, and will make sure that your plate is full of them during the six-week plan later in the book, but for now know those twelve key nutrients are:

- **Folate.** This nutrient is not only important for expectant mothers, but it also helps support the creation of new cells. This B vitamin can be found in foods like beef liver, brussels sprouts, oranges, and leafy greens.
- **Iron.** The brain needs red blood cells to function at the highest level. The body uses iron to build hemoglobin, an important protein in those red blood cells that helps transport oxygen

from the lungs to the brain. You can find iron in pumpkin seeds, oysters, and spinach.

- **Long-chain omega-3 fatty acids.** These long-chain polyunsaturated fatty acids, including eicosapentaenoic acid (EPA) and docosahexaenoic acid (DHA), are made in small amounts by the body, but also must be ingested through the foods you eat. These fatty acids are commonly found in seafood, including wild salmon, anchovies, and oysters.
- **Magnesium.** Magnesium helps to regulate several important neurotransmitters, including those that facilitate mood. It's also known to improve sleep quality. This mineral is found in almonds, spinach, and cashews.
- **Potassium.** Potassium is needed for every electric impulse that travels along a neuron. Many fresh fruits and vegetables contain this essential mineral, including bananas, broccoli, sweet potatoes, and white beans.
- **Selenium.** Selenium helps create a powerful antioxidant in your brain and is necessary for proper functioning of the thyroid gland, which is involved in regulating mood, energy, and anxiety. Mushrooms, Brazil nuts, and oatmeal contain this mineral.
- **Thiamine.** Thiamine, also known as vitamin B1, is fundamental to brain health because of its role in energy production. It's found in beef, nuts, and legumes.
- **Vitamin A.** Several studies have now linked vitamin A to neuroplasticity, or the brain's ability to grow and adapt in response to the environment. Liver, mackerel, and wild-caught salmon are high in vitamin A.
- **Vitamin B6.** Vitamin B6 plays a pivotal role in brain development and function. It's found in whole grains, pork, and eggs.
- **Vitamin B12.** Vitamin B12 is central to your production of mood-regulating brain chemicals serotonin, norepinephrine, and dopamine and supports the myelination of brain cells,

helping to transmit signals more efficiently and effectively. Clams, beef liver, and mussels are foods that are high in B12.

- **Vitamin C.** Vitamin C is a powerful antioxidant that can counteract the damage caused by free radicals in brain cells. Cherries, chiles, and mustard greens are all foods that can get you vitamin C outside of your daily orange juice.
- **Zinc.** Zinc is another mineral that helps to regulate brain signaling and neuroplasticity. Adding pumpkin seeds, oysters, and ground turkey to your diet can help increase your zinc levels.

We will talk about all these nutrients, and a few more, in greater detail in the following chapters. But, instead of focusing on eating more of a particular nutrient or this year's trending "superfood," I want to focus on expanding your diet to include more food categories, or different groupings of foods that hold high brain nutrient density. While it's easy to concentrate on a singular superfood—I'm not known as a "kale evangelist" for nothing—we all have different tastes when it comes to what we put in our mouths. By looking more broadly at food categories, you will soon see that many of these essential nutrients tend to travel together. And it's possible to eat to beat depression and anxiety without ever having to take a single bite of kale.

Moving forward, I will highlight all the ways these different food categories can help support peak brain health—and explain why increasing your intake of these nutrient-rich foods can help prevent depression. We will also discuss why fiber, good bacteria, and anti-inflammatory foods can also aid in this fight. But as we continue to talk about these nutrients, as well as their anti-inflammatory and microbiome-nourishing properties, in the following chapters, I want to be clear on a powerful and simple fact: food is a mental health factor that is entirely within your control. At the end of the day, you choose which nutrient-dense options are best for you. And you should choose the ones you consider most joyful and delicious.

Food is medicine. The field of Nutritional Psychiatry is showing us, study by study, that mental health is largely dependent on the foods you eat. As such, by making some targeted, evidence-based changes to your current diet, adding in nutrient-dense foods that can provide the building blocks your brain needs to thrive, you have the power to improve your mental health. In the next few chapters, we'll discuss the latest science about how your diet can affect your brain in a variety of different ways. Scientists are learning that there are vital nutrients that can help you prevent or manage depression and anxiety. And they do so by fostering a better, stronger, and more dynamic brain. Let's get started.

CHAPTER 1: Recap

- Over the past few years, physicians across the globe have discovered that food plays a key role in preventing and managing physical health conditions, including cardiovascular disease and diabetes.
- The emerging field of Nutritional Psychiatry is a new and growing movement focused on the use of nutrition to optimize brain health and, in doing so, help prevent and treat mental health concerns.
- The *Diagnostic and Statistical Manual of Mental Disorders* (DSM-5), the diagnostic tool used by psychiatrists, defines depression as a person having multiple symptoms, which may include a depressed mood, loss of energy, diminished ability to concentrate, changes in appetite, and decreased interest or pleasure in normally enjoyable activities, for more than a two-week period. It also states that depression is disruptive, meaning that a person's decreased mood is interfering with their ability to comfortably live their lives.
- The DSM-5 defines generalized anxiety disorder, the most common anxiety disorder, as "excessive anxiety or worry," with symptoms that may include feeling "keyed up," irritability, fatigue, and sleep troubles. To be diagnosed with anxiety, you would be experiencing some of those symptoms more days than not over a six-month period.

- To highlight the foods that contain the highest concentration of brain-boosting nutrients that can help with depression, my colleague Laura LaChance, MD, and I created the Antidepressant Food Scale (AFS). It includes folate, iron, long-chain omega-3 fatty acids, magnesium, potassium, selenium, thiamine, vitamin A, vitamin B6, vitamin B12, vitamin C, and zinc.
- Anxiety is greatly impacted by nutrition. While a lot of research has focused on depression, nutrition plays a huge role in regulating anxiety. While depression and anxiety are different conditions, there is a large overlap in the foods and lifestyle choices that will benefit both, because these interventions improve brain health.
- Research studies are demonstrating that diets, like the Mediterranean-style diet, that are full of such nutrients have the power to prevent and manage mental health conditions like depression and anxiety.

Chapter 2

TWELVE NUTRIENTS FOR A BETTER BRAIN

The Brain's Essential Building Blocks

Have you ever stopped to consider what your brain is made of?

Often, we talk about the brain as a muscle. You've likely heard some expert or other tell you that your brain, much like the muscles in your body, needs mental exercise to stay healthy. Use it or lose it, they say—encouraging mental stimulation to help your brain grow faster, stronger, and, overall, stay fighting fit. Both brains and muscles contain special fibers that help them function. And, of course, after a hard workout, like a final exam or a tough crossword puzzle, your brain may feel as fatigued as your legs do after maxing out your mileage on the treadmill.

It's an easy analogy to throw into everyday conversation, the sort of comparison that helps to inspire people to engage in intellectual challenges like Sudoku puzzles or book clubs—and it also does a fair job of highlighting how the brain can change and improve over time.

That said, the brain doesn't actually resemble a muscle in the slightest.

The brain is the most complex organ in the human body. This three-pound command and control center contains more than

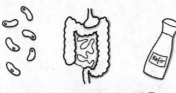

THE MICROBIOME

The trillions of bacteria in the gut
that regulate the immune system
and influence mental health.

THE NEW DEPRESSION

INFLAMMATION

The immune system's response to stress.

High brain inflammation is part of
depression and anxiety.

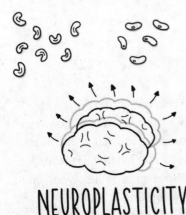

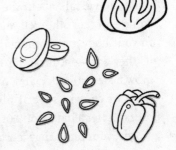

NEUROPLASTICITY

The process of birth, growth, and maintenance
of brain cells by neurotrophins like BDNF.

eighty billion neurons, the special cells that transmit nerve impulses and form the synapses, or key connections, that facilitate every thought, feeling, and action. The brain also houses another category of unique cells, called glial cells, that make up the fatty, insulating sheath surrounding neurons. Some experts estimate there are likely three times the number of glial cells as neurons— and their unique makeup allows them to indirectly improve the efficacy and efficiency of neural signaling across the cortex. The

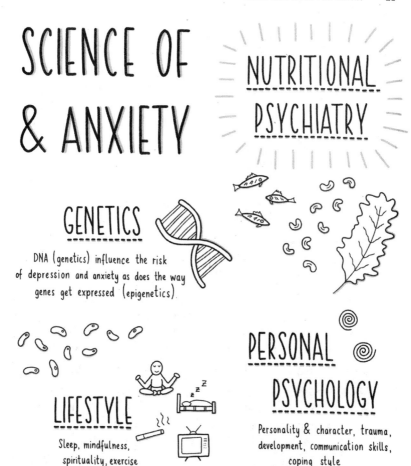

SCIENCE OF & ANXIETY

NUTRITIONAL PSYCHIATRY

GENETICS

DNA (genetics) influence the risk of depression and anxiety as does the way genes get expressed (epigenetics).

LIFESTYLE

Sleep, mindfulness, spirituality, exercise

PERSONAL PSYCHOLOGY

Personality & character, trauma, development, communication skills, coping style

fibers those neurons and glial cells make are quite different, both in terms of form and function, than the sorts of fibers you find in the muscles.

While the brain may already seem quite crowded with those billions upon billions of cells, it's also home to a host of blood vessels and capillaries, which provide brain cells with the rich, oxygenated blood they need to thrive. You can also find a cornucopia of different signaling molecules, including hormones and neurotransmitters that help pass neural messages from cell to cell. You've likely heard about neurotransmitters like serotonin, dopamine, and glutamate—all of which have been implicated in depressive and anxiety disorders. Scientists have also found that signaling molecules like NMDA, glutamate, and endocannabinoids play a role, too. That said, I shouldn't forget to mention the cell receptors. These are distinct proteins that "catch" the signaling molecules, allowing messages to travel from cell to cell at the synapse.

Admittedly, there's a lot to keep track of here—and I've only just scratched the surface of the contents of this extraordinary organ, as well as all the ways each constituent may interact with another to promote optimal brain health. (Note: In the following chapter we will talk about an additional brain molecule, called brain-derived neurotrophic factor [BDNF], which many neuroscientists refer to as a form of "brain fertilizer.")

But now that we've outlined the basics, what I want you to understand about your brain is that what you eat, and your brain's overall well-being, will always be intimately connected. And that's because, simply put, your brain is made of food.

Our brains consume 20 percent of everything we eat—and those foods provide the energy and nutrients to produce and support each element that makes up our brains. Those critical neurotransmitters and receptors? They're made from specific proteins and amino acids that you consume through food. Similarly, the condition of your glial cells is dependent on getting enough omega-3 fats. Minerals like zinc, selenium, and magnesium not only provide the building blocks to form cells and brain tissue but also help to synthesize vital neurotransmitters. B vitamins have been shown to aid in conducting nerve impulses. When the brain is deprived of one or more of these brain-healthy nutrients, cognition, mood, and overall function will ultimately suffer. Take serotonin, the neurotransmitter linked to mood. Without eating foods that contain adequate levels of nutrients like iron, folate, and vitamin B12, your body cannot produce adequate levels of this mood-enhancing chemical.

Historically, we've put minimal thought and focus into how food choices relate to our brains. But it doesn't have to be that way. You can dictate what sort of building materials you want to provide your brain. You can eat these very high-quality, nutrient-dense ingredients and foods to help your brain work at its highest level. When it does, you are in a place to better prevent and manage mood and anxiety disorders.

Ultimately, you, and only you, have the power to decide what you'd like your brain to be made of—and, in doing so, put your brain into a mode of growth, resilience, and health. Truly, better brains are made, not born, by the decisions you make about the foods you consume every day.

THE CHANGING FOOD LANDSCAPE AND ITS EFFECT ON MENTAL HEALTH

Over the past century, the way we eat has changed dramatically. Our great-grandparents nourished themselves with fresh, seasonal, whole foods, grown and nurtured on farms located within a dozen miles from their homes. Today, the American "foodscape" is built on the foundation of industrialized farming operations and pre-packaged items. Nearly 60 percent of what we consume falls into the processed food category, with its correspondingly excessive levels of refined carbohydrates and sugar, food dyes, trans fats, and preservatives. You can't drive more than a few blocks without passing a fast food joint or convenience store. The types of foods that are most accessible—and being actively marketed to you and your family—are full of the very ingredients your doctors are strongly warning you to avoid.

When I first became interested in the intersection of food and mental health, I learned a lot about how, over the past few decades, the average American dietary pattern has changed. Instead of dairy fats, we were told it was better to eat vegetable oils and margarine. They were easy and inexpensive to produce—and, unlike dairy products, have a long, stable shelf life. With that one change, a tremendous amount of trans-unsaturated fatty acids, or trans fats, which we now know to be linked to heart and brain disease, became a staple of the typical Western diet. We have changed the color of foods, adding in unnatural dyes with carcinogenic properties. Processed foods, to maintain their flavor and texture, are preserved with high amounts of sodium and sugar. Look at the ingredient labels of many packages in the grocery store and you'll likely see more chemicals than actual food ingredients. Not only does this make it harder for us to eat the nutrients that can help us beat depression and anxiety—essential nutrients we best get through consumption of the foods that contain them—but the typical Western diet also has us taking in a number of nutrients and molecules that are actually detrimental to brain health. Because of that, most of us are increasing our risk of developing depression or anxiety through the everyday foods we eat.

Something's got to give.

These modern changes to the food supply have markedly altered the way we nourish our bodies. Instead of getting vital nutrients found naturally in whole foods that provide the building blocks for healthy brains, we are instead getting a host of chemicals and preservatives. While our stomachs may be sated by these convenience foods, our brains remain hungry. The vast majority of Americans, according to the United States Department of Agriculture (USDA), aren't meeting the Recommended Daily Allowance (RDA) for key nutrients—about one-third of us are lacking zinc, 68 percent are deficient in magnesium, and a whopping 75 percent aren't getting enough folate. Our brains will struggle to function at their best if they can't get the basic elements they need to flourish.

How do I know this? While it is something that I, and many of my colleagues in the emerging field of Nutritional Psychiatry, have long presumed, our suspicions are now supported by an abundance of new converging evidence. There are a large number of research studies that demonstrate that what we eat is directly associated with our mood and anxiety levels.

THE INTERSECTION OF FOOD AND BRAIN HEALTH

Nearly sixty years ago, epidemiological studies (studies that look at health and disease trends within specific populations of people) discovered something rather interesting. Individuals who lived in Mediterranean nations, like Spain, Greece, and Italy, were less likely to suffer from heart disease than those in other parts of the world. Scientists were very interested to understand why. Was it the importance of family and community to the culture? Regular physical exercise? The food? All of the above?

Over decades of research attempting to answer those very questions, researchers soon realized that all of these factors were important to health and well-being as we age. But, in looking more deeply at dietary patterns, they also observed that the Mediterranean way of eating, which is typically high in fresh fruits and vegetables, seafood, whole grains, nuts, and olive oil, was not only good for your heart but also good for your brain. Study after study showed this diet was instrumental in reducing the risk of heart attack and stroke—and as the researchers delved deeper into the data, they also noticed eating in the Mediterranean style was linked to a decrease in the incidence of dementia and depression.[1,2] Previous studies have shown that regular olive oil consumption, in and of itself, helps prevent depression, as well as reduce the severity of symptoms in those who have been diagnosed with it. But it appears that healthy fat does not work alone. The Mediterranean diet's focus on whole foods, grains, and seafood is also important for maintaining health and well-being.

It's important to note that the Mediterranean diet's effects aren't limited to the senior citizen crowd, either. One of my favorite epidemiological studies, called the SUN Navarra study, was conducted at Spain's University of Navarra. The researchers followed 10,094 former university students, none of whom reported experiencing feelings of depression or taking antidepressant medications at the start of the study, to investigate the role of diet in the later development of a depressive disorder. As you may know, the late teenage and early adulthood years are often when people first start to struggle with depressive symptoms. If we could come up with targeted interventions to prevent depression, this would be an outstanding time to do it.

At the beginning of the study, the researchers gave each study participant a food questionnaire to assess what kinds of foods they ate on a regular basis. That survey contained 136 questions to help the researchers better characterize each person's dietary pattern—and better understand the frequency with which they consumed common Mediterranean diet foods, like fresh vegetables, seafood, whole grains, and healthy fats. Next, a trained dietician analyzed those results and assigned each person a Mediterranean diet adherence score. The more the person ate in the Mediterranean style, the higher their score would be.

The researchers found that the study participants who had the highest adherence scores were much less likely to develop depression over the nearly four-and-a-half-year period. In fact, they found that those who ate in this manner had a 42 percent reduced risk. It's probably not much of a surprise to learn that the study participants who ate more of a Western-style diet, full of simple carbohydrates, vegetable oils, and processed foods, saw their likelihood of developing depression move in the other direction. They were at a higher risk of a mood disorder. These results fall in line with the decades of previous studies that show that the Mediterranean diet can help shield us from heart and brain disease. In this case, what the University of Navarra researchers saw was that strong adherence to this diet protected individuals from depression.

This sort of epidemiological study has now been replicated a number of times, across a variety of different populations varying in age, sex, and location. When you put them all together, the results have profound implications for ways in which we might decrease the burden of depression. We can do so by preventing depressive episodes from ever occurring. That said, it's important to note that the Mediterranean lifestyle includes more than just food. People who live in Greece and Italy do consume a lot of olive oil—but they also tend to walk, bike, and swim more than their average American counterparts. In fact, the SUN Navarro study noted that study participants who had higher Mediterranean diet adherence scores also tended to be more physically active. Might there be any evidence to suggest changing only dietary patterns might affect mood?

As it so happens, there is. Psychiatrists at the University of Pittsburgh Medical Center (UPMC) conducted a lifestyle intervention study with older adults who had previously struggled with depressive episodes. They recruited ninety-five participants, aged fifty or older, to receive dietary coaching to modify what they ate to be healthier. Ironically, at first, these psychiatrists did not think dietary coaching would make a lick of difference; they just wanted some sort of healthy, positive intervention to compare to other forms of talk-based psychotherapy to see which would best serve older patients who were not keen on taking an antidepressant.

The dietary coaching these psychiatrists used wasn't very complicated. In fact, the researchers just gathered some general advice from various government agencies for a nurse or mental health counselor to review with the participants during six to eight sessions. The interventionists shared general nutritional guidelines, reviewed food intake, and helped participants create meal plans and grocery lists to make it easier to follow the diet. The coaching sessions weren't very long, either. The introductory session lasted about an hour, but the subsequent sessions were only about thirty minutes each. On average, each participant received only about eight hours of coaching across two or three months. The UPMC researchers were therefore shocked to discover that participants who received dietary coaching experienced a 40 to 50 percent improvement in their depressive symptoms over the course of the study. Even more impressive is that those improvements stuck around for more than two years. Given that most analyses suggest that talk therapy shows an incidence rate reduction of between 20 and 25 percent for depression, the UPMC results are something to celebrate.

The UPMC researchers were quick to state that their study cannot provide direct evidence that changing your diet can reduce depressive symptoms—even though several other nutrition intervention studies have now come out with similar results. To establish a causal relationship, meaning demonstrating that a particular intervention results in a particular outcome, you need what's called a clinical randomized controlled trial. This type of study, where people are chosen at random to receive a type of clinical intervention to compare to a control, is one of the most powerful tools you can find in clinical research. It's the gold standard for testing any treatment. Any Food and Drug Administration (FDA) approved drug, for medical conditions ranging from eczema to cancer, has been through this kind of rigorous testing.

Since the UPMC study was not a randomized trial—and as admitted by the researchers, they never intended to study dietary coaching as a treatment option—it's possible there may be some other factor, at least in part, that explains the improvement in depressive symptoms seen in this study. It became clear that it was high time to have a clinical trial to see whether dietary interventions were as effective as we were beginning to believe they were.

There is plenty of data to show that diet matters when it comes to depression and anxiety. In fact, in a recent analysis undertaken by researchers from the University of Delhi in India, the authors concluded that there is growing and substantial evidence of a relationship between diet quality, nutritional deficiencies, and mental health, making it an obvious place where psychiatrists and mental healthcare providers could make changes to prevent or manage mental health conditions like depression.[3] But without a clinical trial, that "gold standard" for testing a treatment, it's been hard to definitively argue that mental health professionals should be prescribing dietary changes to their patients struggling with depression and anxiety.

FINALLY, THE GOLD STANDARD IS HERE

For decades, psychiatrists have relied on antidepressants and psychotherapy to help manage depression and anxiety. Lifestyle factors, including diet, were all but ignored. But, then, in 2017, researchers from Australia's Mood and Food Centre at Deakin University School of Medicine published the first randomized, controlled clinical trial of a dietary intervention for adults with major depressive disorder. It was aptly named the SMILES study (Supporting the Modification of lifestyle In Lowered Emotional States).

This research, led by two leaders in the field of Nutritional Psychiatry, Felice Jacka and Michael Berk, recruited 176 participants suffering from depression, many of whom were already receiving treatment in the form of medication or talk therapy. Half were randomly assigned to a dietary intervention that involved seven individual nutrition consulting sessions with a certified dietician. Each session lasted approximately an hour and occurred over a period of three months—and the dietician spent that time educating each person about the Mediterranean diet and helping participants to adopt a modified version of the plan. A lot of it really was just helping these patients make some smart swaps or additions— switching out butter for olive oil or new ways to add more legumes to their favorite meals. The other half of the study participants were given a control condition, a "befriending" protocol where, instead of dietary information, the interventionists spent the same amount of time basically just visiting with participants.

"There was a large amount of data pointing to this connection between food and mental health, but correlation does not necessarily mean causation. We needed to test whether changes in diet could affect depression," Jacka said. "That's why we decided to do the study."

Developing a clinical trial around dietary interventions is no easy task. You cannot, for example, assign one group to a "junk food" diet for comparison. It wouldn't be ethical. Thus, Jacka and colleagues decided on using the befriending protocol to compare to the dietary advice group.

"This kind of befriending protocol is often used in psychotherapy trials because it's like going to see a psychotherapist or other health practitioner, except you don't receive the counseling," she said. "You are getting a face-to-face interaction with someone. You still have someone who will listen and talk to you for an hour—and we know that kind of connection is helpful for people with depression."

The researchers took a baseline measure of depressive symptoms for each participant at the start of the study—and then again three and six months later. They discovered the individuals in the dietary group had a remission rate of approximately 32 percent. Think about that: about one-third of the people who received a dietary intervention completely remitted from depression. The researchers controlled for nearly every other factor. This was not a matter of social interaction or exercise—though, admittedly, both are important in the prevention and treatment of mental health conditions, too. It wasn't a matter of weight loss, either. Study participants' weight did not significantly change over the trial. It really came down to small but lasting changes to diet. Since then, other trials have shown similar results: dietary changes can help to reduce or even remit depressive symptoms.[4]

"We didn't think diet would have such a big impact—we thought it would be much more subtle," Jacka said. "All our dieticians did was educate patients on what they should be eating and give them some advice on how to get there by making small changes. There were so many stunning things that came out of this trial, but I think, one of the biggest is that people could improve their diet even though they had clinical depression at the moderate to severe level. They were able to make changes and incorporate more healthful foods into their diet despite their symptoms. Second, we saw quite a substantial difference in remission. Roughly 30 percent of those who were in the dietary intervention went into what we call clinical remission, which means their depression scores were at a level where they would no longer be considered clinically depressed."

Jacka added there was a tight association between the degree to which people improved their diet and the degree to which their depressive symptoms improved.

"The more people were able to improve their diet, the better off they were," she said. "It was quite remarkable."

Put it all together and what we see is that food matters. These are extraordinary results—and ones that have direct bearing on how we, as mental health practitioners, could amend our treatments to both empower our patients and better manage their depression in the future.

But what about anxiety? Does the SMILES trial have any bearing on those symptoms? When asked, Jacka said examining diet's effect on depressive symptoms was their primary purpose—but they saw a decrease in anxiety, too.

"Anxiety was a secondary outcome for us—we were focused on depression," she said. "But the people in the dietary group also showed significant improvement in measures of anxiety symptoms compared to those who participated in the social support group."

While this was a small trial, several studies have now replicated Jacka's findings, including a 2019 intervention study done by Heather Francis and colleagues at Australia's Macquarie University that showed similar results in young adults. Francis recruited 101 young adults, aged seventeen to thirty-five, with active symptoms of depression and a not-so-great dietary pattern to undergo a three-week intervention. Half of the participants received a diet intervention via a thirteen-minute video, which they could access and rewatch as needed, featuring a registered dietician offering tips on how to adhere to a Mediterranean-style diet and encouraging them to increase their intake of veggies, whole grains, nuts, fish, and olive oil. They also received a small basket of some of these foods to help them get started and brief phone calls at the end of weeks one and two to gauge how they were doing. The other half were given no instructions regarding diet and were simply asked to return in three weeks.

Francis, like Jacka, found that individuals who received guidance on how to improve diet reported significantly lower depression and anxiety symptoms after three weeks—as well as three months later when the researchers followed up with each with a phone call.[5] Francis wrote that she was surprised that not only could the depressed participants make such positive changes to their diets, but the effects also lasted months longer than the study. In fact, 70 percent of the students maintained several important aspects of the dietary advice. It just goes to show—diet matters, and matters a lot, when it comes to brain health.

These randomized, controlled trials demonstrate that changing diet has the power to change mental health. By replacing junk foods with those that contain brain-boosting nutrients, you can find ways to improve your brain's overall health and function.

CREATING THE ANTIDEPRESSANT FOOD SCALE (AFS)

My colleague Laura LaChance, MD, is a fellow psychiatrist and clinical researcher at the University of Toronto Centre for Addiction and Mental Health. Like me, this deluge of evidence regarding the importance of diet to mental health inspired her, so we decided to take a deeper dive together. We understood that simply telling patients to eat in the Mediterranean style wasn't enough. When you are feeling depressed or anxious, it can be difficult to make lifestyle changes—though, as Jacka found, it can be done. To make it even easier for clinicians and patients, we wanted to pinpoint exactly which nutrients the scientific literature suggested had the most power to combat depression and which foods had the most of these nutrients. That way, instead of telling patients to simply follow the Mediterranean diet to the letter, we could recommend particular food categories that contained the most necessary nutrients to promote brain health.

(At this moment, you may be saying to yourself, "Wait! I already take a multivitamin supplement every morning. Isn't that enough?" To be honest, I hear that kind of thing a lot. I'll talk about this more in Chapter 6, but the long and the short of it is that supplements aren't the be-all and end-all when it comes to getting the right nutrients for your body and brain. The body was designed to absorb vital nutrients from food. Supplements simply can't compete.)

To identify the nutrients that best support brain health, and the food categories that contain them, Dr. LaChance and I combed the available scientific literature to rank all the research regarding essential vitamins and minerals linked with preventing and treating depression. From this we were able to create a new nutritional scale you might remember from Chapter 1 called the Antidepressant Food Scale. This scale ranks the foods that are most nutrient dense and full of the different vitamins and minerals to best combat depression and, most likely, anxiety, too. Dr. LaChance and I highlighted not only the essential nutrients that can help optimize mental health but also the foods in which you can find them. These are the vitamins, minerals, and other molecules that help to optimize brain structure and function.

WHAT ARE THE ESSENTIAL NUTRIENTS TO EAT
TO BEAT DEPRESSION AND ANXIETY?

Folate

The human body needs folate, also known as vitamin B9, to make and regulate DNA, as well as to make major neurotransmitters we know are strongly linked to depression like serotonin and dopamine. Neurotransmitters are special signaling chemicals that help brain cells communicate with one another. Healthy brains are chock-full of these molecules, helping to ensure that cells can do their jobs, whether it's to perceive what's happening in the world around you or regulate your mood.

You've likely heard of folate before—it's commonly prescribed to pregnant women to support spinal cord and brain development in the fetus. It's probably not a surprise then that what's good for fetal brain development also supports overall brain health in adults. Folate helps to regulate your mood, your ability to experience pleasure, and your ability to think clearly.

Folate is the natural form of folic acid. The word folate comes from *folium*, the Latin word for "foliage"—which gives you an easy reminder of one place you can find this vitamin: in leafy greens. Because of its role in building critical brain molecules and supporting processes, low levels of folate can result in low mood, low energy, and feelings of worry. We check the blood level of folate as part of the medical workup for clinical depression as studies have found up to one-third of depressed patients are deficient.

A lack of adequate folate has also been linked to increased levels of inflammation. Folate helps to break down a special amino acid called homocysteine. This amino acid is a general marker of inflammation in the body. Without enough folate to metabolize homocysteine, levels will rise—and high homocysteine is a serious risk factor not only for depression but also heart disease.

Food Categories: *Leafy Greens, Rainbows, Beans*

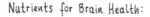

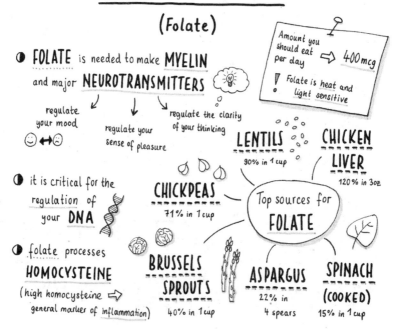

Nutrients for Brain Health:

VITAMIN B9

(Folate)

- **FOLATE** is needed to make **MYELIN** and major **NEUROTRANSMITTERS**

  regulate your mood

  regulate your sense of pleasure

  regulate the clarity of your thinking

  Amount you should eat per day ⇒ 400 mcg

  Folate is heat and light sensitive

- it is critical for the regulation of your **DNA**

- folate processes **HOMOCYSTEINE** (high homocysteine ⇒ general marker of inflammation)

Top sources for **FOLATE**

LENTILS 90% in 1 cup

CHICKEN LIVER 120% in 3oz

CHICKPEAS 71% in 1 cup

BRUSSELS SPROUTS 40% in 1 cup

ASPARGUS 22% in 4 spears

SPINACH (COOKED) 15% in 1 cup

Iron

The brain requires approximately 20 percent of your energy to effectively function—and to create that energy, your brain cells need unfettered access to hemoglobin, the iron-based protein in your blood that transports oxygen from the lungs to the brain, and myoglobin, another iron-based protein that stores oxygen in the muscles for when you need a burst of energy. That is why many argue iron is the nutrient most critical to overall brain function.

It also plays a role in the development and management of depression and anxiety. Beyond helping the brain get the oxygen it needs, iron is also a needed factor in the production of two key neurotransmitters responsible for regulating mood, focus, and pleasure—

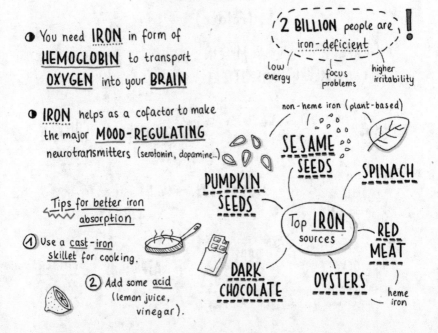

Nutrients for Brain Health:

IRON

- You need **IRON** in form of **HEMOGLOBIN** to transport **OXYGEN** into your **BRAIN**

- **IRON** helps as a cofactor to make the major **MOOD-REGULATING** neurotransmitters (serotonin, dopamine...)

2 BILLION people are iron-deficient !
low energy   focus problems   higher irritability

Tips for better iron absorption

1. Use a cast-iron skillet for cooking.
2. Add some acid (lemon juice, vinegar).

non-heme iron (plant-based)
SESAME SEEDS
SPINACH
PUMPKIN SEEDS
Top **IRON** sources
RED MEAT
DARK CHOCOLATE
OYSTERS
heme iron

dopamine and serotonin. Like folate, iron is also an ingredient of myelin, the fatty insulating material that makes your neurons capable of ultrafast signal conduction.

Given the importance of this nutrient, it's easy to understand why low levels of iron have been linked to brain fog, decreased energy levels, and poor mood. Iron demand is of particular concern for vegetarians, as the iron available in plants is 30 to 40 percent less absorbable than the iron you find in meat and seafood. You can increase absorption by adding an acid like lemon juice or vinegar or using a cast-iron skillet.

Food Categories: *Seafood; Nuts, Beans, and Seeds; Leafy Greens; Meat*

Nutrients for Brain Health:

OMEGA-3 FATS

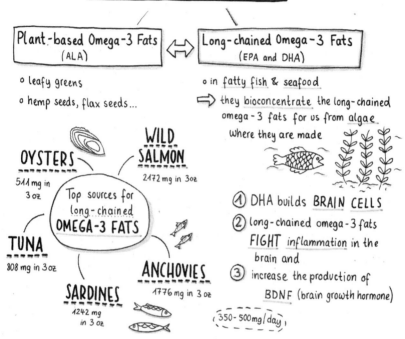

Plant-based Omega-3 Fats (ALA) ⟷ Long-chained Omega-3 Fats (EPA and DHA)

○ leafy greens

○ hemp seeds, flax seeds...

○ in fatty fish & seafood

⟹ they bioconcentrate the long-chained omega-3 fats for us from algae where they are made

OYSTERS
511 mg in 3 oz

WILD SALMON
2172 mg in 3 oz

Top sources for long-chained **OMEGA-3 FATS**

TUNA
808 mg in 3 oz

ANCHOVIES
1776 mg in 3 oz

SARDINES
1242 mg in 3 oz

① DHA builds **BRAIN CELLS**

② long-chained omega-3 fats **FIGHT** inflammation in the brain and

③ increase the production of BDNF (brain growth hormone)

(350-500mg/day)

Long-Chain Omega-3 Fatty Acids

These special long-chain polyunsaturated fats (PUFAs) are amazing brain boosters and have made headlines over the past few years for good reason. They're the longest and most complex fats that you can eat, stimulating the brain to produce more of important nerve growth factors that promote neuroplasticity, or the ability for your brain to grow and change. They've also been implicated in regulating—and reducing—inflammation levels in the brain and body.

It's important to understand that not all omega-3s are created equally. There are actually two types of omega-3 PUFAs: the shorter, less complex plant-based omega-3s, which you may have heard referred to as alpha-linolenic acid (ALA); and the more complex omega-3 fats like eicosapentaenoic acid (EPA) and docosahexaenoic acid (DHA). While plant-based omega-3s have numerous health benefits and are an essential part of any diet, to really eat to beat depression and anxiety, you want to make sure you have adequate levels of the more complex kind as well.

EPA helps promote brain function by lowering the concentration of pro-inflammatory molecules in your brain cells. DHA, on the other hand, helps to make up cell membranes and, as such, plays a vital role in synaptic function, facilitating the connections between your brain cells. DHA is estimated to compose about 8 percent of the dry weight of your brain. In addition, DHA also plays an anti-inflammatory role, acting as a building block for important hormones called neuroprotectins and resolvins. Human brains, particularly those that are still developing, benefit from a diet rich in these fats. A lack of adequate omega-3 PUFA consumption has been consistently associated with depression, as well as a host of other brain disorders.

Food Category: *Seafood*

Magnesium

Magnesium, sometimes called the "calming chemical," plays a leading role in an astounding number of body processes. When it comes to the brain, this macromineral is required for the proper function of nerve and brain cells, helping to promote synaptic transmission and neuromuscular conduction. In fact, magnesium is one of the few nutrients that directly stimulates brain growth. It's been implicated in hundreds of different chemical reactions that occur in a healthy body and is one of those basic ingredients in your brain's chemistry that affects functions ranging from the production of DNA to the efficient disposal of cellular waste.

Magnesium was one of the very first nutrients shown to help treat depression. Numerous studies have identified a connection

Nutrients for Brain Health:

MAGNESIUM

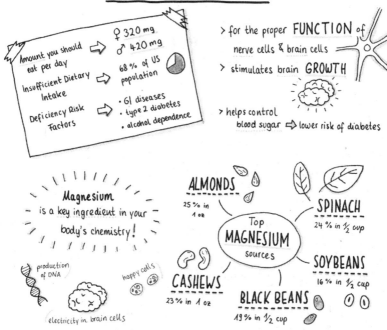

Amount you should eat per day ⇒ ♀ 320 mg ♂ 420 mg

Insufficient Dietary Intake ⇒ 68 % of US population

Deficiency Risk Factors ⇒ · GI diseases · type 2 diabetes · alcohol dependence

> for the proper FUNCTION of nerve cells & brain cells

> stimulates brain GROWTH

> helps control blood sugar ⇒ lower risk of diabetes

Magnesium is a key ingredient in your body's chemistry!

production of DNA

happy cells

electricity in brain cells

ALMONDS 25 % in 1 oz

Top MAGNESIUM sources

SPINACH 24 % in ½ cup

SOYBEANS 16 % in ½ cup

CASHEWS 23 % in 1 oz

BLACK BEANS 19 % in ½ cup

between magnesium deficiency and poor mood. But, all the way back in 1922, when a group of patients with "agitated depression" were given an IV infusion of magnesium, they were observed to be calm and feeling better—many of them were even observed to be sleeping—only a few hours later. Since then, studies have repeatedly shown that low magnesium levels increase the risk for depression.

I think about magnesium as a way to conduct the flow of energy from the sun all the way to your brain; it's the mineral at the center of photosynthesis. That's why a dietary pattern that's rich in plant-based foods is so important. The main source of magnesium is within those fruits, vegetables, and leafy greens; it's one of the very first minerals I think of when a patient tells me about their diet.

Food Categories: *Leafy Greens; Nuts, Beans, and Seeds; Rainbows*

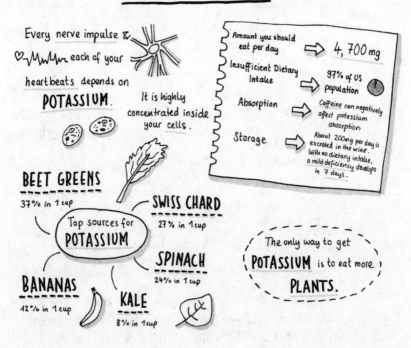

Nutrients for Brain Health:

POTASSIUM

Every nerve impulse & ♡~M\/M~ each of your heartbeats depends on **POTASSIUM**.

It is highly concentrated inside your cells.

Amount you should eat per day ⟹ 4, 700 mg

Insufficient Dietary Intake ⟹ 97% of US population

Absorption ⟹ Caffeine can negatively affect potassium absorption

Storage ⟹ About 200mg per day is excreted in the urine. With no dietary intake, a mild deficiency develops in 7 days.

BEET GREENS
37% in 1 cup

SWISS CHARD
27% in 1 cup

Top sources for **POTASSIUM**

The only way to get **POTASSIUM** is to eat more **PLANTS**.

SPINACH
24% in 1 cup

BANANAS
12% in 1 cup

KALE
8% in 1 cup

Potassium

This mineral enables every nerve impulse and every neural signal across the human nervous system. Scientists have long understood that potassium helps cells remain in homeostasis, or healthy balance, by allowing the cell membrane to pump in vital nutrients and pump out waste. As such, it plays a role in getting oxygen to the brain and relaying signals from neuron to neuron.

A lack of adequate potassium has been linked to mental fatigue, as well as a decrease in mood. Potassium also helps to regulate serotonin levels, while low levels have been implicated in chronic pain. A 2008 study found that a high-potassium diet, made up of mostly plant-based foods, helped to alleviate symptoms of depression.[6]

Food Categories: *Rainbows, Leafy Greens*

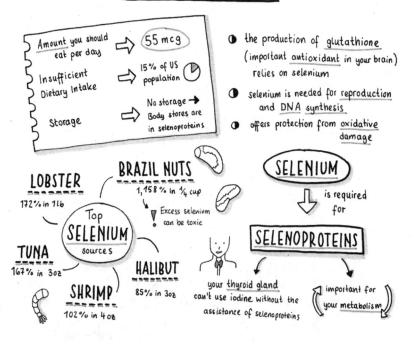

Nutrients for Brain Health:

SELENIUM

Amount you should eat per day ⟶ 55 mcg

Insufficient Dietary Intake ⟶ 15% of US population

Storage ⟶ No storage → Body stores are in selenoproteins

- the production of glutathione (important antioxidant in your brain) relies on selenium
- selenium is needed for reproduction and DNA synthesis
- offers protection from oxidative damage

Top SELENIUM sources

LOBSTER
172% in 1 lb

BRAZIL NUTS
1,158% in ¼ cup

Excess selenium can be toxic

TUNA
167% in 3 oz

HALIBUT
85% in 3 oz

SHRIMP
102% in 4 oz

SELENIUM

is required for

SELENOPROTEINS

your thyroid gland can't use iodine without the assistance of selenoproteins

important for your metabolism

Selenium

Antioxidants help protect cells, including brain cells, from damaging, inflammatory molecules called free radicals. The most powerful antioxidants are not the ones you eat, but the ones your own body makes. In order to make those antioxidants, however, the body needs the appropriate ingredients. Selenium is one of those. Glutathione is the top antioxidant in the brain and is important to helping keep brain cells working their best.

This mineral also plays an important role in regulating metabolism, DNA synthesis, and brain signaling pathways. It is critical to thyroid health. It's probably not a surprise that a deficiency in selenium has been linked to both depression and anxiety.

Food Categories: *Rainbows, Seafood*

Nutrients for Brain Health:

VITAMIN B1 (Thiamine)

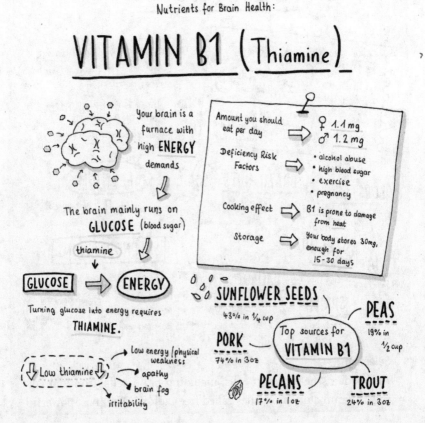

Your brain is a furnace with high **ENERGY** demands

The brain mainly runs on **GLUCOSE** (blood sugar)

thiamine

GLUCOSE ⟹ **ENERGY**

Turning glucose into energy requires **THIAMINE.**

⬇ Low thiamine ⬇
→ Low energy / physical weakness
→ apathy
→ brain fog
→ irritability

Amount you should eat per day ⟹ ♀ 1.1 mg ♂ 1.2 mg

Deficiency Risk Factors ⟹
• alcohol abuse
• high blood sugar
• exercise
• pregnancy

Cooking effect ⟹ B1 is prone to damage from heat

Storage ⟹ Your body stores 30mg, enough for 15-30 days

SUNFLOWER SEEDS 43% in ¼ cup

PORK 74% in 3oz

Top sources for **VITAMIN B1**

PEAS 19% in ½ cup

PECANS 17% in 1oz

TROUT 24% in 3oz

Vitamin B1

We've already discussed that the brain has immense energy needs. Like the rest of the body, the brain gets that energy from glucose. In order to transform glucose to energy, the brain needs adequate levels of thiamine, also known as vitamin B1.

Vitamin B1 was the very first vitamin to be discovered and isolated by scientists. Individuals who are severely deficient in B1 develop beriberi, a disease that negatively affects the cardiovascular system, eventually leading to severe neurological and psychiatric symptoms since the brain can't get the energy it needs to

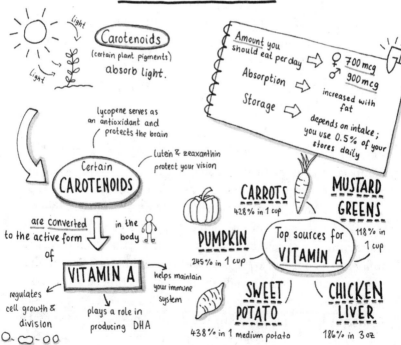

function. While most will never lack thiamine to the point of developing beriberi, less than optimal levels have been linked to symptoms including low energy, apathy, brain fog, and irritability.
Food Categories: *Seafood, Leafy Greens, Rainbows*

Vitamin A

This vitamin, sometimes referred to as retinol, is found in meat, eggs, and dairy. You also make retinol by converting the color pigments of plants, mainly bright orange and yellow vegetables that contain carotenoids. Vitamin A molecules not only work as antioxidants, helping to prevent cellular damage due to inflammation, but also help to regulate cell growth and division. Vitamin A also plays a role in the body's ability to produce DHA, that long-chain omega-3 fatty acid, which is a key constituent of brain health. Several studies have now suggested that ample consumption of vitamin A is strongly linked to a reduced risk of dementia, cancer, and depression. Even newer research also suggests that vitamin A helps to facilitate neuroplasticity, or the brain's ability to form new synapses and adapt in response to the environment.
Food Categories: *Rainbows, Meat, Eggs*

Vitamin B6

Vitamin B6, also called pyridoxine, is another member of the B vitamin family. Its main responsibility is to help convert the food we eat into energy. It also plays a pivotal role in how the nervous system functions, from early development on through adulthood.

Vitamin B6 is one of the ingredients required to make neurotransmitters like serotonin and norepinephrine, both of which influence mood. It also helps create melatonin, the hormone that regulates the body clock and tells us when it's time to sleep. With its other vitamin B family cousins, it also helps to decrease levels of homocysteine—and, therefore, inflammation—as well as to make the red blood cells that help port oxygen to the brain. When B6 is

Nutrients for Brain Health:

VITAMIN B6

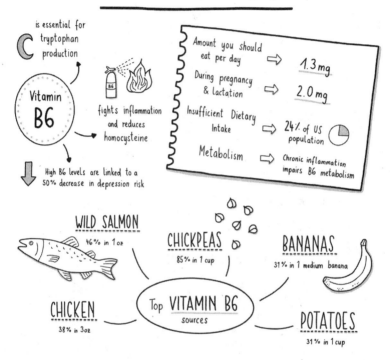

is essential for tryptophan production

Vitamin B6

fights inflammation and reduces homocysteine

High B6 levels are linked to a 50% decrease in depression risk

Amount you should eat per day ⇒ 1.3 mg

During pregnancy & lactation ⇒ 2.0 mg

Insufficient Dietary Intake ⇒ 24% of US population

Metabolism ⇒ Chronic inflammation impairs B6 metabolism

WILD SALMON
46% in 1 oz

CHICKPEAS
85% in 1 cup

BANANAS
31% in 1 medium banana

CHICKEN
38% in 3oz

Top VITAMIN B6 sources

POTATOES
31% in 1 cup

low, people often have trouble concentrating. They may also experience feelings of nervousness, irritability, and sadness.

Food Categories: *Seafood, Rainbows, Beans, Meat*

Vitamin B12

Like the other B vitamins, vitamin B12 (cobalamin) helps to produce crucial brain chemicals that regulate mood and anxiety levels, including serotonin, norepinephrine, and dopamine. In addition, it also supports the myelination of brain cells, which, as we've discussed,

Nutrients for Brain Health:

B12

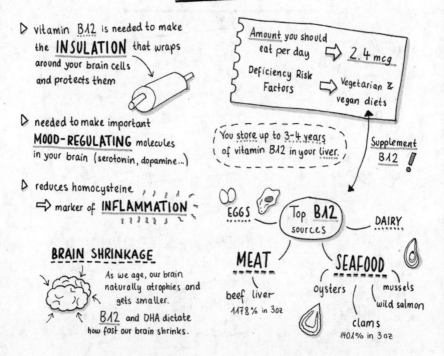

▷ vitamin B12 is needed to make the **INSULATION** that wraps around your brain cells and protects them

▷ needed to make important **MOOD-REGULATING** molecules in your brain (serotonin, dopamine...)

▷ reduces homocysteine ⇨ marker of **INFLAMMATION**

Amount you should eat per day ⇨ 2.4 mcg

Deficiency Risk Factors ⇨ Vegetarian & vegan diets

You store up to 3-4 years of vitamin B12 in your liver.

Supplement B12 !

BRAIN SHRINKAGE

As we age, our brain naturally atrophies and gets smaller.

B12 and DHA dictate how fast our brain shrinks.

Top **B12** sources

EGGS

DAIRY

MEAT

beef liver 1178% in 3oz

SEAFOOD

oysters

mussels

wild salmon

clams 1401% in 3oz

allows synaptic messages to travel across the brain more efficiently. Like B6, it also helps to decrease homocysteine. Approximately 10 to 15 percent of adults over the age of sixty are deficient in this vitamin, which, unfortunately, increases their risk of developing a depressive disorder.

A previous randomized controlled trial showed that vitamin B12 supplements assisted in treating depressive symptoms in patients who had been diagnosed with major depressive disorder. But individuals can get ample vitamin B12 from a well-balanced diet that includes foods like eggs, milk products, and bivalve seafoods like clams and mussels.

Food Categories: *Seafood (especially bivalves), Meat, Eggs and Dairy*

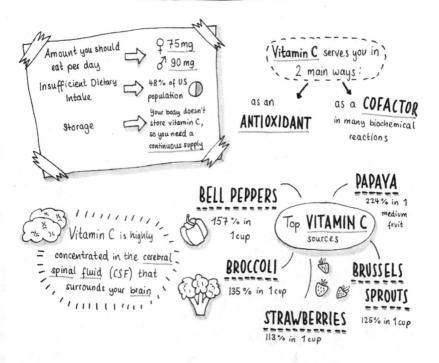

Nutrients for Brain Health:

VITAMIN C

Amount you should eat per day → ♀ 75mg ♂ 90 mg

Insufficient Dietary Intake → 48% of US population

Storage → Your body doesn't store vitamin C, so you need a continuous supply

Vitamin C serves you in 2 main ways:

as an **ANTIOXIDANT**

as a **COFACTOR** in many biochemical reactions

Vitamin C is highly concentrated in the cerebral spinal fluid (CSF) that surrounds your brain

Top **VITAMIN C** sources

BELL PEPPERS 157% in 1 cup

PAPAYA 224% in 1 medium fruit

BROCCOLI 135% in 1 cup

BRUSSELS SPROUTS 125% in 1 cup

STRAWBERRIES 113% in 1 cup

Vitamin C

Vitamin C doesn't just help prevent colds. This powerful anti-oxidant helps to counter the damage caused by inflammatory processes in both the body and the brain. It also acts as a cofactor in many chemical reactions and, in doing so, promotes cell health and neural signaling. It also can help you better absorb other vital nutrients like iron. There's a reason besides taste behind why we squeeze lemon on our seafood; it helps our bodies get more iron from those fish, clams, and oysters.

We've long known that vitamin C deficiency can lead to scurvy, a disease that features swollen, bleeding gums and issues with wound healing. But not getting enough vitamin C in your diet can also lead to feelings of fatigue and depression. Some studies have shown that increasing vitamin C levels not only helps individuals to better manage depressive symptoms but also to lower anxiety levels.

Food Categories: *Rainbows, Leafy Greens*

Nutrients for Brain Health:

ZINC

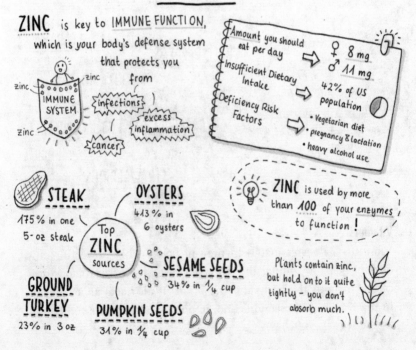

ZINC is key to IMMUNE FUNCTION, which is your body's defense system that protects you from

infections
excess inflammation
cancer

zinc
zinc
IMMUNE SYSTEM
zinc

Amount you should eat per day ➡ ♀ 8 mg ♂ 11 mg

Insufficient Dietary Intake ➡ 42% of US population

Deficiency Risk Factors ➡
• Vegetarian diet
• pregnancy & lactation
• heavy alcohol use

STEAK 175% in one 5-oz steak

OYSTERS 413% in 6 oysters

Top **ZINC** sources

SESAME SEEDS 34% in ¼ cup

GROUND TURKEY 23% in 3 oz

PUMPKIN SEEDS 31% in ¼ cup

ZINC is used by more than 100 of your enzymes to function!

Plants contain zinc, but hold on to it quite tightly – you don't absorb much.

Zinc

This important mineral plays a role in cellular processes and immune function. It's a protective nutrient, helping to support your body's natural defense systems to fight medical conditions like cancer, infections, and excess inflammation. It's also involved in the regulation of synaptic transmission and neuroplasticity. Low zinc levels are difficult to measure. But the result can lead to lowered levels of key neurotransmitters like glutamate and serotonin, increasing your risk of depression and anxiety.

Food Categories: *Nuts and Seeds*

OTHER KEY PLAYERS

When Dr. LaChance and I identified the twelve nutrients above, our focus was on finding those that could best help our patients eat to beat depression. That said, most of these nutrients are also instrumental in preventing and managing anxiety disorders. As I've said before, depression and anxiety often travel together. By eating the nutrient-dense foods that support overall brain health, you should find some relief for anxiety—as well as a host of other mental health issues. Studies have certainly suggested that omega-3s, as well as B vitamins, all are important in the fight against anxiety symptoms.

There is, however, another nutrient that's been directly implicated in anxiety. Choline is a special molecule (another member of the B-vitamin family) that's important to the synthesis of lipids, including the myelin that insulates your neural circuitry. It's a brain builder that makes phosphatidylcholine, the most common fat in all cells and helps to regulate inflammation. It's also a key ingredient of an important neurotransmitter, acetylcholine, that's important to learning and memory.

Anxiety is often described as a learning process gone awry, so making sure you have enough choline to support learning and

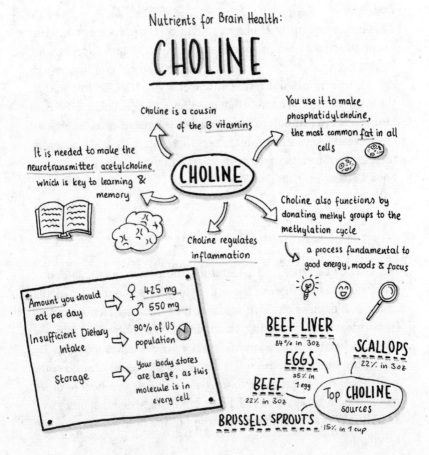

Nutrients for Brain Health:

CHOLINE

Choline is a cousin of the B vitamins

You use it to make phosphatidylcholine, the most common fat in all cells

CHOLINE

It is needed to make the neurotransmitter acetylcholine which is key to learning & memory

Choline also functions by donating methyl groups to the methylation cycle

a process fundamental to good energy, moods & focus

Choline regulates inflammation

Amount you should eat per day	⟹	♀ 425 mg, ♂ 550 mg
Insufficient Dietary Intake	⟹	90% of US population
Storage	⟹	Your body stores are large, as this molecule is in every cell

BEEF LIVER
84% in 3oz

SCALLOPS
22% in 3oz

EGGS
35% in 1 egg

BEEF
22% in 3oz

Top **CHOLINE** sources

BRUSSELS SPROUTS
15% in 1 cup

memory can help get those processes back on track. The Hordaland Health Study of 4632 adults suggests individuals who consume more choline, usually through eggs, are less likely to develop an anxiety disorder.

I'd also be remiss if I didn't mention phytonutrients—good fats, and good bugs—as other nutrients to recruit in your fight for optimal brain health. Phytonutrients, the molecules and nutrients that come from "eating the rainbow," or a wide assortment of colorful fruits and vegetables, help to promote neurogenesis,

Nutrients for Brain Health:

MONOUNSATURATED FATS

(MUFAs)

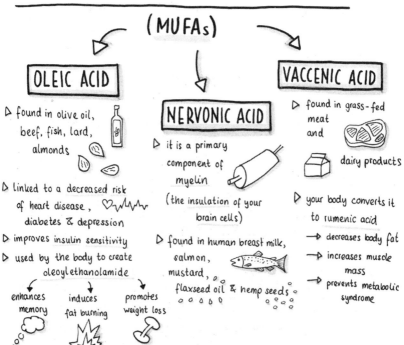

OLEIC ACID

▷ found in olive oil, beef, fish, lard, almonds

▷ linked to a decreased risk of heart disease, diabetes & depression

▷ improves insulin sensitivity

▷ used by the body to create oleoylethanolamide

enhances memory

induces fat burning

promotes weight loss

NERVONIC ACID

▷ it is a primary component of myelin (the insulation of your brain cells)

▷ found in human breast milk, salmon, mustard, flaxseed oil & hemp seeds

VACCENIC ACID

▷ found in grass-fed meat and dairy products

▷ your body converts it to rumenic acid

→ decreases body fat
→ increases muscle mass
→ prevents metabolic syndrome

or the development of new brain cells, as well as reduce inflammation. Monounsaturated fatty acids (MUFAs), like those found in the olive oil so prevalent in the Mediterranean diet, also fight inflammation—as well as provide the building blocks for myelin and cell membranes.

And then there are the good bugs, the healthy bacteria that naturally live within our guts. You may not realize that you've been populating your gut with these healthy bacteria since you were a baby. Everything you've touched—and everything you've eaten—

has helped to determine which species live there. In Chapter 4, we'll learn more about the best ways to get more of these good bugs, but for now what I want you to know is that these microorganisms play a role in regulating mood, improving cognition, and decreasing anxiety levels. All of these, along with the twelve nutrients, are fundamental players in eating to beat depression and anxiety.

CHANGING PATTERNS, IMPROVING MENTAL HEALTH

My goal is to help you fuel your brain and in turn beat your anxiety and depression. But I also understand that each of us has our own tastes, values, and requirements when it comes to deciding what foods we want to fill our plates. Later, we'll focus on the different food categories that contain one or more of these brain-boosting nutrients to better guide you as you think about ways you might incorporate them into your diet. Whether you're a strict vegetarian or are following a keto diet, there are many ways to eat to beat depression and anxiety.

While it would be easy to tell you to focus on eating more zinc or one of these brain-healthy nutrients—or even to just go out and spend some money on some supplements—I understand it's not a joyful way to eat or interact with food. I'm not trying to tell you your dietary pattern is bad or wrong, but rather that there are places where you can make improvements to bolster your mood and better keep those worrying thoughts at bay. I've addressed these nutrients here to help you understand how they affect brain health and, consequently, your mood and anxiety levels.

Your brain is not a muscle—but it was designed to thrive and grow when it can get the right nutrients. In the next chapters we'll discuss why bigger, healthier brains are built from the foods that fight inflammation and promote brain health at any age—and why nurturing your brain with such foods can help you in your quest to prevent or manage depression or anxiety.

CHAPTER 2: Recap

- The brain is the most complex organ in the human body, containing tens of billions of neurons, as well as other key cells and support molecules.
- Our brains consume 20 percent of everything we eat—and the foods we eat provide the energy and nutrients to produce and support each element that makes up our brains.
- Modern changes to the food supply have markedly changed the way we nourish our bodies. Instead of getting vital nutrients found naturally in whole foods that provide the building blocks for healthy brains, we are instead getting a host of chemicals and preservatives.
- While a number of epidemiological studies have hinted at the relationship between food and mental health, it was only recently that the first randomized, controlled clinical trials looking at dietary interventions were published.
- The results from both these types of studies are clear: food has the power to improve mental health, preventing conditions like depression and anxiety, as well as help to alleviate symptoms after they've been diagnosed.
- These were the studies that inspired Dr. LaChance and me to develop the Antidepressant Food Scale (AFS)—and start putting it into practice with patients.
- Studies have shown that the key nutrients on this scale support brain development and maintenance in a variety of vital ways.

. . . .

Chapter 3

HOW TO GROW NEW BRAIN CELLS

How Your Food Choices Affect Brain Growth

Over the past few decades, psychiatry and neuroscience have learned a great deal about the biological underpinnings of depression and anxiety. Large-scale genetic studies, called genome-wide association studies, have discovered that a significant portion of patients with these conditions share similar genetic features. We now understand there are certain gene variants, often tied to different neurotransmitters or receptors, that can increase a person's likelihood of developing depression or anxiety. Understanding mental health in this detailed way is important—and we hope it will help doctors like me better select more specific, targeted treatments to help our patients better manage depression and anxiety.

These studies have been instrumental in helping patients understand that depression or anxiety is not some sort of personal failing or inability to cope with life. Rather, these conditions are, at least in part, biological—not just situational. But knowing this can also make some patients feel a little more hopeless about finding relief.

Remember Pete? When he first came to see me, he had moved back in with his parents and couldn't find any work. During our very first meeting, he told me he felt "stuck in place." The word "stuck" stood out for me. Because Pete wasn't only talking about having to move back into his childhood bedroom. He was talking about how it felt for him to live with depression.

"Sometimes I think it doesn't matter what I do, I'm always going to feel like this," he said.

Pete had been diagnosed with depression as a teenager. He'd been taking an antidepressant medication for a number of years, but it didn't seem to be working as well for him anymore. Understandably, that was very frustrating. He wasn't the only person in his family to have dealt with depressive episodes, either. He worried at times that, thanks to that family history, his brain was somehow "broken," and his genes meant that he'd always be struggling with these feelings of sadness and decreased motivation.

Pete's not the only patient I've seen who felt this way. Many who struggle with depression and anxiety feel like they've been dealt a bad hand when it comes to their genes. That's understandable. For too many years, we've talked about our DNA in terms of biological destiny. When I was finishing medical school nearly twenty years ago, we believed that an individual's genes strictly determined everything from intelligence to behavior. The core message was that our genomes are directly responsible for how our bodies grow, mature, and function. And whatever configuration of genes you happened to be born with was all you had, and would ever have, to work with.

We thought similarly about the brain. Back then, common wisdom held that once you reached adulthood, your brain was done developing and maturing. Your genes had dictated how it would grow and once it was done, it would stay in that same state, barring insult or injury, for the rest of your life. You can see, with that kind of messaging, why Pete and others might feel "stuck" after a mental health diagnosis. If depression or anxiety is solely due to a malfunctioning brain, built off a faulty genetic blueprint, it's difficult to feel like you can do all that much to make a difference.

As it turns out, we were completely off the mark. Today, with another decade or two of genetic research under our belts, we acknowledge that our brains are fully capable of change across the life span. We know that genes play an important role in determining how our brains work, of course—but they don't work in a vacuum. The emerging field of epigenetics, the study of how our environments and lifestyle decisions can change where, when, and how our genes are expressed, is showing us that biological destiny is much more malleable than we ever imagined.

An easy way to conceptualize epigenetics is to think of your genome as a desktop computer. You were born with your genome, made up of all the DNA passed to you by your mother and your father, with a few mutations or tweaks in your genes thrown in along the way. There may even be a few genes that predispose you to depression or anxiety. But, as with your computer, the hardware needs software to tell it what to do. The epigenome, or those environmental tweaks to gene expression, is that software. Your life experiences, as well as lifestyle factors like diet, exercise, and social interactions, are actually marking up your DNA—and telling the genome to increase, decrease, or even stop production of different proteins in response to interactions you have with your environment. It's complex, of course—but what we see is that, even with a strong family history of a particular mental health condition, nothing is set in stone. The epigenome means that you have the power to make changes, like to your diet, that can counter and check what may have built into your brain's hardware since birth.

The other great thing about this emerging field is that it has shown us that our brains are neuroplastic—that is, they harbor the ability to grow and adapt to our environments no matter our age. That means no one is ever "stuck." Each and every one of us has the power to make changes, including more educated decisions about what we eat, to modify the way our genes are expressed, and help move our bodies and brains into a place where we can better manage depression and anxiety.

NEUROPLASTICITY

Your brain in ✦GROW✦ mode

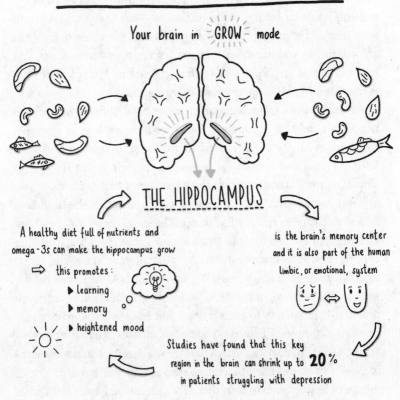

THE HIPPOCAMPUS

A healthy diet full of nutrients and omega-3s can make the hippocampus grow

➡ this promotes:
- ▶ learning
- ▶ memory
- ▶ heightened mood

is the brain's memory center and it is also part of the human limbic, or emotional, system

Studies have found that this key region in the brain can shrink up to **20**% in patients struggling with depression

BIGGER BRAIN, BETTER BRAIN

As we discussed in the last chapter, there have been several studies that show a strong relationship between the quality of a person's diet and their mental health status. Individuals who eat a more Mediterranean-style diet are not only more likely to prevent the development of depression or anxiety, but, if they do happen to be diagnosed with it, following that kind of whole-food dietary pattern can help them better manage their symptoms. The open question, then, is how diet helped. What was diet doing to the brain to influence mood in this manner? Felice Jacka, director of the Food and Mood Centre at Australia's Deakin University, and the researcher who led the SMILES trial, decided to take a look at the hippocampus to see if it might provide any clues.

"The hippocampus is a key center of learning and memory in the brain, but we also know that this area is involved in mental health," said Jacka. "We aren't sure exactly how, but neuroimaging studies show that people with depression have a smaller hippocampus. When they are successfully treated for depression, their hippocampus grows."

You've probably heard of the hippocampus before. This small, seahorse-shaped region is often described as the brain's memory center. It also happens to be a part of the human limbic, or emotional, system—and, as such, is also affected by mood and anxiety disorders. In fact, studies have found that this key region, which is critical to learning and memory, can shrink as much as 20 percent in patients who are struggling with depression. That's a pretty significant change and one, perhaps, that could shed some light on the relationship between diet and depression.

Jacka stated that knowledge, paired with fascinating work coming out of Fernando Gomez-Pinella's lab at the University of California Los Angeles contradicting the idea that adult brains could not foster the growth of new brain cells, inspired her to investigate the relationship between diet and hippocampal volume.

"This groundbreaking work from Dr. Gomez-Pinella's lab was showing evidence of neurogenesis, or the birth of new neurons, in the hippocampus in animal models," she said. "They saw that the growth of new cells, as well as the shrinkage of the hippocampal area, was very much predicated by neurotrophins, or the proteins that prompt the growth of neurons. These studies showed you could manipulate the levels of these important proteins and that brain growth by manipulating diet."

When Gomez-Pinella's group fed rats foods chock-full of nutrients and brain-supporting omega-3s, they saw that the hippocampus grew—and the rats showed improved cognition and mood. Given all this converging data showing a link between diet, neurotrophins, and hippocampal volume, Jacka and colleagues decided to directly examine the relationship between the way people eat and hippocampal size as measured by volume. They asked 255 individuals, aged sixty to sixty-four, to fill out a questionnaire to assess their dietary practices. They then took brain scans of each person, once at the beginning of the study and then again after four years, to look at diet's effect on the hippocampus. They found individuals who ate healthier were more likely to have a larger hippocampal volume. Those who partook in the unhealthier "Western" dietary pattern showed the opposite effect. Jacka said they were not surprised by the results.

"Based on the extensive animal work showing this link, I was not shocked to see a very clear relationship between diet and hippocampal volume. Those with better diet quality had a substantially increased hippocampal volume," she said. "This wasn't a trivial association—and it was independent of all these other factors that we thought might be relevant."

This study, once again, suggests there is a relationship between dietary pattern and mental health. Since then, two other larger studies have replicated Jacka's results and shown that diet quality matters. Bigger hippocampi are stronger hippocampi, with a greater number of more-connected cells that are reaching out and communing with their neighbors in order to promote learning, memory, and heightened mood. Bigger hippocampi are healthier hippocampi, chock-full of the brain chemicals and molecules that facilitate its ability to work with the rest of your brain at the highest possible level. When you put this evidence together with the clinical trials that have tested diet and mood, what we see is that diet can play an important role in the prevention and treatment of mental health conditions. And it's a role, of course, that mental health practitioners can no longer ignore. Jacka agreed.

"What we see is there is a negative impact of poor diet on the brain and brain function," she said. "As we've seen more and more work from animal studies, observational studies, and neuroimaging studies—and triangulated that with what we know about biology—it becomes clear that diet is an area where we can intervene to promote brain growth and brain function."

The brain is a vibrant and dynamic organ. It's an organ of connection. When it's getting the nourishment it needs, it can move into what I call "grow mode"—a place that facilitates neuroplasticity, allowing it to easily make the strong new synaptic connections required to better adapt to the world around you. That "grow mode" also happens to be a protective state, producing the defensive molecules that help to safeguard your brain against the atrophy that is so often seen in mood disorders.

THINKING BEYOND SEROTONIN—MEET BDNF

If I asked you to name a brain chemical that plays an important role in mental health, particularly in depression or anxiety, what would it be? There's a good chance you'd say serotonin. It's not a surprise. Scientists have linked an imbalance in this vital neurotransmitter to both depression and anxiety—and the most commonly prescribed type of antidepressant medication, selective serotonin reuptake inhibitors (SSRIs), works by increasing the levels of serotonin floating around the synapse. When it comes to mood and anxiety disorders, serotonin has definitely gotten the lion's share of attention over the past few decades. But new research now stresses the role of another brain chemical called brain-derived neurotrophic factor, or BDNF for short.

BDNF is what's called a neurotrophic factor or a neurotrophin—

one of those important brain-growing proteins that Jacka mentioned. It's a special protein, widely expressed across the central nervous system, that supports the growth and survival of brain cells. Some say BDNF is a lot like Miracle-Gro for the brain—a fertilizing biomolecule that supports the birth of new brain cells and synapses during development. It's an apt nickname. But BDNF also plays a key role in helping to keep our brains healthy, whole, and adaptable in adulthood, giving our brains that little something extra they need to make new synaptic connections. In fact, in the laboratory, when you sprinkle a little BDNF on a sample of brain cells, you can actually watch those cells reach out and form new connections with neighboring cells. It's quite something to see.

BDNF, however, is much, much more than just fertilizer. It's also a protective molecule. When your brain is exposed to toxins— like the trans fats found in certain foods or the hormones your body produces in response to chronic stress—your brain cells have to work a little harder not only to form the synaptic connections required for a healthy brain but also just to survive. In fact, they need all the extra help they can get. BDNF provides that help, making your brain cells more resilient in the face of those threats. It allows them more room to adapt and grow in the face of whatever may be happening in the world around you. Taken together, you can see why having ample amounts of BDNF flowing in the brain is important to its overall health and well-being, facilitating the growth and survival of strong, resilient, and connected brain cells.

The opposite also holds true. When BDNF is lacking, the brain can and does suffer. There have now been numerous studies that show that patients with major depressive disorder and anxiety disorder have lower BDNF levels than those without such diagnoses. The expression of the BDNF gene, which makes this vital brain-fertilizing protein, is somehow downregulated in these conditions. The gene simply isn't producing as much BDNF as you'd see in a healthy brain. In addition, studies have also demonstrated that a particular variant of the BDNF gene, called the Val66Met

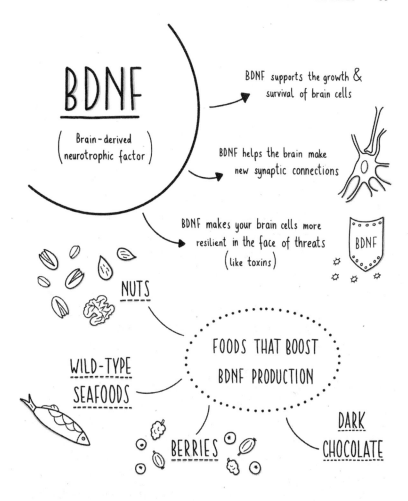

BDNF

(Brain-derived
neurotrophic factor)

BDNF supports the growth &
survival of brain cells

BDNF helps the brain make
new synaptic connections

BDNF makes your brain cells more
resilient in the face of threats
(like toxins)

BDNF

NUTS

WILD-TYPE
SEAFOODS

FOODS THAT BOOST
BDNF PRODUCTION

BERRIES

DARK
CHOCOLATE

polymorphism, seems to make those that have it more challenged by stressful life events and childhood adversity.[1] In these cases, when the going gets tough, the BDNF faucet decreases to a small drip—which, ultimately, can lead to the development of depression or anxiety.

You might think, with all this talk of biomolecules and gene variants, we're back to that old "stuck" argument—but again, genes are not destiny. You can increase the amount of BDNF your body produces, regardless of any Val66Met polymorphisms. And you can do so by eating foods that bolster the production of BDNF, like nuts and leafy greens. The power to make your brain more resilient in the face of stress really does lie at the end of your fork.

Numerous animal studies conclude that the right diet can increase BDNF production—and also create other key neurotrophic factors. But researchers from Spain's University of Las Palmas de Gran Canaria also showed it in human beings. In the PREDIMED-NAVARRA trial, these groundbreaking researchers wanted to see if certain foods, added to your everyday diet, could increase the production of BDNF. As you're already aware, numerous studies have now shown that the Mediterranean diet can improve depressive symptoms. But are there certain foods within the typical Mediterranean diet that can increase BDNF—and, by extension, neuroplasticity—to make such improvements?

To test the idea, the researchers took a closer look at 243 patients, aged fifty-five to eighty, who were already enrolled in a larger dietary intervention trial to reduce cardiovascular disease risk. In the larger study, those individuals had already been randomly placed into one of three diet groups: a basic low-fat diet, a Mediterranean diet supplemented with additional virgin olive oil, or a Mediterranean diet with the addition of a daily 1-ounce serving of walnuts, almonds, and hazelnuts. The participants followed their dietary assignment for four years, meeting with a trained dietician for advice every three months. At the end of three years, the researchers compared BDNF levels in each participant to when they started the trial. They discovered that patients who followed the Mediterranean diet had higher BDNF levels than those who simply ate low-fat food. But, astonishingly, those who ate the Mediterranean diet with just that extra daily handful of nuts showed significantly higher levels of BDNF than the other groups. For the patients in the group who had issues with depression at the start of the trial, the jump in BDNF was even higher—with a corresponding drop in depressive symptoms. As it turns out, upping your dietary game in just a single food category—in this case, nuts—can make a dramatic difference.

This suggestion—that adding about an ounce of nuts can make such changes—may surprise you. But not when you consider that, in order to make enough BDNF for optimal brain health, your body needs the ingredients and signals to do so. You need to consume enough of the key amino acids, the building blocks of proteins, as well as essential vitamins and minerals, to up your BDNF levels. Many of those very building blocks are found in nuts. Other foods can help increase BDNF, as well. Studies now show that diets with higher consumption of omega-3 fatty acids from wild-type seafoods, resveratrol in red grapes, zinc in pumpkin seeds and oysters, and anthocyanins from berries can all help boost BDNF production— and, in doing so, can help you eat to beat depression and anxiety.

These foods, however, don't only increase the production of neurotrophic factors. As I said earlier, they're also protective. That extra handful of nuts each day isn't just helping your brain cells foster strong connections across vital circuits. It's also helping to defend your brain cells from damage when bombarded by pro-inflammatory molecules.

INFLAMMATION ABOUNDS

Inflammation is a buzzword in medicine these days—and for good reason. This natural immune response is a very good thing in moderation. When the body suffers injury or illness, the immune system will release a variety of different proteins and hormones, including white blood cells, special cytokines like interleukin-6, or even proteins like c-reactive protein (CRP), to fight off invaders, clear out damaged cells, and help the body heal. You probably noticed inflammation the last time you got a scratch on your arm. In response to the wound, the immune system kicked off the defensive inflammatory processes, which led to some redness and swelling around the injury during the first day or two. Those physical symptoms are signs that the immune processes were doing their jobs.

Issues may arise, however, when inflammation continues to occur for prolonged periods of time. In that case, perfectly healthy cells can be and often are affected. For some reason, and we don't entirely understand why, the immune system gets the wrong message and starts attacking not only the damaged cells but also the normal ones in the near vicinity. When chronic inflammation pairs up with certain genetic susceptibilities, autoimmune diseases like asthma, psoriasis, ulcerative colitis, and rheumatoid arthritis can develop. Over time, the healthy tissues will also start to come under attack from all those different immune molecules—and they can be adversely affected in the process.

The brain, like the rest of the body, can also be affected by inflammation. There are several types of specialized immune cells that help keep the brain in top shape. The first are called astrocytes. These unique star-shaped cells, which are a type of glial cell, are part of the brain's support and cleanup crew. When there is some sort of damage to neurons, like those infections or injuries we talked about, these cells rush to the scene, clean up any damaged cells, and then carry them away.

Another type of glial cell called microglia also takes on a crucial immune role. They are the primary type of immune cell found in the brain, surveying the other cells, including neurons, for signs of trouble. These unique cells circulate, briefly touching each neuron in their path, as if they're just checking in to say hi. If, during that surveying process, everything appears normal, the microglia move on. But, if the microglia interact with a cell that is in some sort of trouble, they are moved to action—either nibbling away at its synaptic connections or consuming the damaged cell so it can be taken out with the rest of the trash. We now understand that both microglia and astrocytes are vital to immune function—and to keeping the brain working its best.

Roger McIntyre, a physician and psychopharmacologist at the University of Toronto, has studied how inflammation can alter brain function. He said it's important to note that inflammation, in and of itself, is not bad—in fact, the inflammation system is actually a "good guy" that helps to keep our bodies and brains in tip-top shape.

"We need the inflammatory system," he said. "While we used to think that microglia only served a simple role as structural support for neurons, we now understand they have an important immune function, going through the brain, pruning different connections, and even removing cells. This cleansing process is necessary for the brain to evolve and develop properly. The inflammatory system helps with that."

But factors like chronic stress, environmental toxins, or hormone imbalances, just to name a few, can lead to an imbalance in the release of pro-inflammatory and anti-inflammatory molecules— with too many pro-inflammatory chemicals let loose in the brain. And that's when trouble can start.

"When there's an imbalance, and large numbers of pro-inflammatory molecules flood the brain, it endangers key cells and circuitry," McIntyre explained. "All that inflammation leads to loss of cells, which can affect the neural circuits, and can then affect human experience. When the inflammatory system goes awry, it can lead to a very dangerous situation in the brain—altering neural circuit and neural network activity in select regions of the brain related to arousal, fear, and emotion."

One of those areas that McIntyre references is the hippocampus; it probably doesn't surprise you to learn that dangerous situations are linked to the development of depression and anxiety disorders.

As it so happens, doctors have long observed a curious correlation between the symptoms seen in infection and depression. Think about it: a person with the flu has quite a bit in common with someone with depression. Both tend to have low moods, increased irritability, and a general lack of interest in activities they

typically enjoy doing. They may also present with heightened anxiety symptoms. Those intriguing overlaps raised the question for
psychiatrists as they searched for causes for mental health issues.
We were starting to see that inflammation profoundly affected so
much of the body. Could it be causing problems for the brain, too?

Today, thanks to dozens of groundbreaking studies, we now
understand that chronic inflammation does have a hand in depression and anxiety disorders. In fact, many studies have now
shown that approximately one-third of patients diagnosed with
depression have high levels of different inflammatory markers,
like CRP or interleukin-6, coursing through the body. And when
those inflammation levels are up in the brain, over time, you will
see serious consequences. In fact, when researchers from Emory
University scanned the brains of depressed individuals with high
levels of CRP, they found less activation in key circuits connecting
the brain's reward areas to those responsible for executive function. It's almost like that same swelling you see around a cut in
your arm, only occurring in the brain—and it significantly slows
down the ability of different regions to coordinate and talk to one
another, resulting in common depressive symptoms.[2]

McIntyre said this makes a lot of sense from an evolutionary
standpoint. Thousands of years ago, when humans were surviving
as hunter-gatherers out on the savanna, having pro-inflammatory
molecules push these sorts of symptoms could be an advantage to
survival.

"Back then, typically you'd have an infection or a wound, so altering these different brain systems makes some sense," he said.
"You are very vulnerable in this state, so decreasing motivation and
increasing fear or anxiety could not only help you stay in one place
so you can rest, save your energy, and heal up."

While to date, the majority of studies have looked at the relationship between inflammation and depression, there has been quite a
bit of work showing that pro-inflammatory molecules can alter the

circuitry in the brain's fear centers, too—meaning chronic inflammation has also been reliably linked to anxiety.

"Anxiety is fear—fear of something, whether it's a fear of spiders or a fear of social judgment," said McIntyre.

Once again, thinking about this from that evolutionary standpoint, having a heightened sense of fear can help keep you alive when you are experiencing inflammation after an injury or illness. It can allow you to remain hypervigilant, despite not being at your best, so you can avoid predators or other dangers. That said, in today's modern world, the environment is vastly different—which is why the body producing all that extra anxiety is more harmful than helpful to our day-to-day survival. McIntyre said that fear is, in and of itself, pro-inflammatory—which means all that persistent and pervasive worrying too often can lead to even more persistent and pervasive worrying. You can understand why it's so important to find reliable ways to put this powerful immune response back in balance.

COULD IT JUST BE A SIDE EFFECT?

Over the years, some have argued that inflammation is merely a side effect of depression or anxiety instead of the cause. It's likely that, as McIntyre said, these conditions can add to the release of more pro-inflammatory molecules, leading to a vicious cycle. But that doesn't mean you can't find ways to right the ship, allowing for a more balanced immune response. In fact, a new meta-analysis shows that treating the inflammation in concert with a mood disorder can make traditional antidepressant medications work even better.

Researchers from Aarhus University in Denmark scoured the available literature for clinical trials where patients received antidepressants while also taking a nonsteroidal anti-inflammatory drug (NSAID) or a statin, which are commonly prescribed for conditions like arthritis or high cholesterol levels. You see, it's very common for people with depression to have other physical health problems. Remarkably, many of these physical health issues are also exacerbated by high levels of pro-inflammatory molecules.

But when these Aarhus researchers dug into these studies, many of which actually looked at outcomes for other health issues but took measures of depressive symptoms, they discovered something quite interesting. The addition of these anti-inflammatory agents significantly improved patient mood outcomes—seemingly improving the antidepressant treatments themselves. Reducing the inflammation not only helped to improve the other health problems but also helped to reduce the depression. That's important.

Another interesting piece of evidence comes from work that shows that Prozac, or fluoxetine, which happens to be one of the most popular SSRI medications prescribed to treat depression, also dampens the inflammatory response in individuals who take it. It's a selective serotonin reuptake inhibitor (SSRI), which works by blocking the ability for neurons to absorb serotonin, leaving more to hang out in the synapse, and regulating synaptic transmission. But this drug also tells those pro-inflammatory molecules to close up shop and get on out of the brain. A variety of animal studies have now shown that Prozac treatment not only improves an animal's affect or mood but also lowers levels of pro-inflammatory cytokines in the body.

Does that mean that everyone should now be prescribed an NSAID with their antidepressant and antianxiety medication? Or that Prozac will work for everyone? Of course not. Each person and their mental health struggles are different. But, as it's become more and more clear that anxiety and depression are partially inflammatory diseases, finding reliable ways to reduce the number of pro-inflammatory molecules released by the immune system seems like an important step in providing the best possible treatment outcomes for patients. To understand how to best reduce those molecules, however, one big question remains: where is all this brain inflammation coming from to begin with?

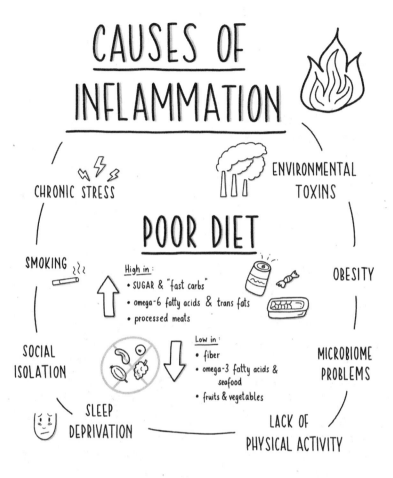

CAUSES OF INFLAMMATION

Unfortunately, when it comes to establishing strict cause and effect here, there is no simple answer. We know there are some reliable culprits: chronic stress, smoking, physical illness, sleep deprivation, environmental toxins, lack of physical activity, social isolation, and obesity have all been consistently linked to increased inflammation in dozens and dozens of research studies. As it so happens, they are all risk factors for mood and anxiety disorders, too. But there's one other offender that keeps popping up in these investigations into the cause of inflammation. If you guessed it was poor diet, you'd be right.

The typical Western dietary pattern—low in fresh fruits and veggies and high in processed meats, refined carbohydrates, and trans fats—has been consistently associated with higher levels of inflammatory markers. People who eat more whole foods–based diets, like the Mediterranean diet, show lower concentrations of those markers. There are many reasons why diet is so closely tied to inflammation. Whole foods–type diets, which promote the consumption of whole grains and phytochemicals, help promote the production of neurotrophins as well as other anti-inflammatory chemicals. Together, these protect our body against the free radicals that are often a consequence of prolonged inflammation. Those healthy cells that are so often "collateral damage" in response to chronic inflammation are better prepared to defend themselves when you are eating plenty of rainbow fruits and veggies with antioxidant properties.

You can also point the finger at convenience foods. We now know that highly processed food made of refined carbohydrates and trans fats promote more of that chronic immune activity. Omega-3 fatty acids, found in food categories such as seafoods and leafy greens, on the other hand, have been repeatedly shown to reduce inflammation. People who regularly consume omega-3-rich seafoods and antioxidant phytochemicals tend to not only have fewer pro-inflammatory molecules coursing through the body and brain—they have a smaller pro-inflammatory response to life's stressors.

Another compelling piece of evidence demonstrating a strong link between inflammation and mental health involves celiac disease, an autoimmune condition caused by an overwhelming inflammatory reaction to gluten. Gluten is a type of protein found in grains like wheat, barley, and rye. When individuals with celiac disease consume gluten, their immune system attacks the lining of the small intestine. Common celiac symptoms are diarrhea, bloating, and fatigue—but a large number of people with celiac disease also report depression and anxiety symptoms. In fact, there's a much higher incidence rate of these mental health conditions in celiac patients.

To better understand the link between celiac disease and mental health, researchers at Rome's Catholic University of the Sacred Heart followed thirty-five patients who had been diagnosed with celiac disease, as well as a group of fifty-nine healthy control participants, for a year after they were prescribed a gluten-free diet. Basically, the study participants were instructed to eliminate wheat and other gluten-containing foods from their diet. That's it.

At the beginning of the study, each person was assessed for both depression and anxiety using standardized measures. Unsurprisingly, those with celiac disease showed both higher levels of depression and anxiety at baseline as compared to those without it. But when the researchers brought the study participants back into the laboratory a year later, they discovered that anxiety, but not depression, had dropped by nearly 50 percent in the celiac group. That's a pretty incredible thing to see. The normal incidence rate of anxiety in the general population is about 20 percent. That means a simple dietary intervention—just removing the inflammatory gluten—had the power to reduce or even eliminate anxiety from this normally hard-hit group.[3]

I mention this study because it shows the role that inflammation can play on mental health. Don't worry—I'm not telling you that you have to give up bread! But people with celiac disease have an innate intolerance for gluten that leads to increased inflammation. And when you can reduce inflammation, your body is in a better position to prevent or manage your anxiety issues. That's huge.

The evidence keeps converging to the same point: the foods you eat can dramatically affect how your body decides to deploy your immune system. When you can find ways to reduce inflammation, your brain—and your mental health—benefit, whether you have an autoimmune condition like celiac disease or not.

INFLAMMATION-FIGHTING NUTRIENTS

The good news is that, just as diet can cause greater bodily inflammation, what you eat can also decrease or even alleviate it. Let me give you two examples of nutrients from the Antidepressant Food Scale that we know can reduce inflammation and, consequently, help you better manage depressive symptoms. The first are omega-3 fatty acids. As I mentioned above, these essential fatty acids, found in wild-type seafoods, help to fight inflammation. They have shown to be effective in reducing depressive symptoms in a number of studies.[4] They also have no known side effects. By substituting seafood for chicken or steak three to four times a week, you can better eat to beat depression and anxiety.

The other nutrient that bears a mention is magnesium. Large-scale epidemiological studies like the Hordaland Health Study, which looked at a population of older adults in Western Norway, have shown that low magnesium levels are not only linked to increased levels of inflammatory markers but also to a higher incidence of depression. Adding magnesium-rich foods, like avocados, dark chocolate, and pumpkin seeds, to your diet can also aid in your fight against depression. Molecular studies now show us that those higher levels of magnesium lead to strengthened synaptic connections, improved sleep, and lower inflammatory cytokine levels—and, by extension, eased mood and anxiety symptoms. The nutrients that help fight depression can also help manage inflammation in the brain's fear and emotional centers and, as a result, help reduce those nagging worries.

If you feel like Pete and so many other people I've encountered—"stuck" because you're battling depression and anxiety—take heart. You're not stuck; you're never stuck. Your brain is a dynamic organ that can always change. You have the power to change it. The scientific evidence now paints a very clear picture—diet matters, and it matters a lot, to both the prevention of depression and anxiety disorders and the successful management of depressive and anxiety symptoms. This is a place where you can make positive changes, opting into a food prescription that will help put your brain into "grow mode" and keep it in a healthier, more balanced state.

While you may not be able to always shut down the extra stress at work or find more hours in the day to sleep, there are always ways to add more brain-boosting nutrients to your diet. With so many intervention studies consistently showing us that moving to a whole foods, nutrient-rich dietary pattern can increase BDNF and decrease dangerous pro-inflammatory molecules, there's no time like the present to start thinking about ways to add more foods from our brain-boosting food categories to your plate.

CHAPTER 3: Recap

- For far too long, we've talked about a person's genetic profile as some sort of biological destiny. We now understand, however, that the brain is fully capable of change across the life span.
- The emerging science of epigenetics, or the study of how our environment and lifestyle decisions can change where, when, and how our genes are expressed, means our choices, like what we eat, can and do influence how well our brains function.
- Studies suggest that a Mediterranean-style diet, chock-full of the nutrients found in the AFS, can put the brain into a "grow" mode—especially in the hippocampus, an area of the brain linked to depression. Individuals who eat a diet rich in seafood, vegetables, and olive oil have larger hippocampi than those who don't.
- While many studies have linked neurotransmitters like serotonin to mental health, there are other neurochemicals that are important. Brain-derived neurotrophic factor is a molecule that acts as both a brain "fertilizer" and as a protectant. A diet high in cashews, walnuts,

almonds, and hazelnuts—as well as omega-3-fatty-acid-containing seafood and anthocyanins in berries—can help make sure your brain has an ample supply of BDNF.

- High levels of inflammation are linked to mental health conditions like depression and anxiety. One of the biggest—and easiest to change—factors that influence an individual's inflammation levels is a poor diet. Diets containing more omega-3 fatty acids, phytonutrients in plants, B vitamins, and minerals such as zinc and magnesium can help keep your levels in check.

. . . .

Chapter 4

OPTIMIZE YOUR GUT FOR MENTAL HEALTH

Depression, Anxiety, and the Microbiome

What if I told you that optimal brain health doesn't just involve your brain? That other parts of your body also help to regulate the neurotransmitters and other neurochemicals that keep your brain in its best shape? It might surprise you—some of the initial studies about this next topic certainly turned the world of psychiatry on its head when they first broke.

As it turns out, significant research studies have now demonstrated that the human gut plays a key role in helping to regulate your mental health. That's right—the gut. Just as there are certain gene variants that can increase an individual's risk of developing depression or anxiety, the constituents of your gastrointestinal tract also contribute to your brain working at its highest level.

When Susan (the busy working mother we talked about in Chapter 1) first came to see me, she wasn't just experiencing heightened anxiety and insomnia thanks to all her life stressors. She was also experiencing fairly serious gastrointestinal (GI) issues. A few years earlier, her primary care doctor had diagnosed her with irritable bowel syndrome (IBS), a condition known for symptoms like cramping, gas, diarrhea, and constipation. As we discussed her medical history, it soon became clear that her stomach pains and diarrhea tended to increase along with her feelings of worry.

"It's just all so embarrassing," she told me. "My stress level goes up and, chances are, you'll find me in the bathroom. Honestly, my stomach issues just end up making me feel even more anxious about things."

Susan's experience is not uncommon. In fact, I started to notice that many of my patients living with anxiety also had some sort of stomach issue that would escalate with their worries. I was seeing it more in my depressed patients, too. There seemed to be a connection between their mental health and their guts. In some ways, it's not a surprise. Humans, as a species, have always regarded the mind and gut as strongly linked. There's good reason that we talk about "gut reactions" and "gut feelings." When we're deeply disappointed or saddened, we're "gutted." And, of course, when we are nervous, like before a big exam or speaking in a large group of people, we tend to feel it in our abdominal regions, maybe as butterflies or as strong feelings of nausea. And though gut issues and mental health have a lot in common, we're only just beginning to understand all the links between them. The symptoms can be challenging and, at times, hard to talk about. In both cases, symptoms are often dismissed by healthcare practitioners, as well as friends and family, as being "all in your head." That's because a lot of these symptoms, which have significant overlap, can be confusing for others to understand.

Over the past century, an extraordinary number of animal studies have shown us that there's bidirectional communication between the gut and the brain. This powerful signaling highway is called the gut-brain axis and it plays an important role in our basic survival. Your GI tract is home to hundreds of millions of neurons that can send messages to the nervous system in a matter of milliseconds. This ability to be in constant communication is an advantage. It can let the brain know that you've eaten to satiety—or that you really shouldn't have indulged in that fourth donut. If you were to eat something disagreeable, such as a toxin or pathogen, the gut can immediately pass messages to the brain about it so it can respond with vomiting or diarrhea to help you rid yourself of the invader. John Cryan, a neuroscientist at University College Cork and one of the authors of *The Psychobiotic Revolution*, said that, simply stated, gut-to-brain communication is vital for homeostasis, or the ability to maintain a stable internal state so your body and brain can work at their best. He likens this bidirectional signaling to the upstairs/downstairs communications that occur in posh houses like the one chronicled in the popular British television show and film *Downton Abbey*. The wealthy owners live in the upstairs of the house, seemingly controlling everything around them, while the servants and staff live downstairs, seeing to the owners' needs.

"The upstairs and the downstairs need each other to survive," he said. "From a distance, it looks like they are completely separate and don't have much to do with one another. But when things start going wrong downstairs that filters to the upstairs. The upstairs can affect the downstairs, too. We see the same when it comes to the gut and the brain."

Even as early as the beginning of the 1900s, scientists could see these effects. At the time, a common approach to treating peptic ulcers was to surgically remove part or all of the stomach in a procedure called a gastrectomy. Doctors who performed this procedure did give those patients some relief from ulcers but, in doing so, they significantly increased their likelihood of developing a psychiatric disorder. Animal studies show similar effects. When you remove parts of the gut and therefore limit the ways the GI tract can communicate with the brain, rats and mice show higher levels of stress, fear-like behaviors, and issues with cognition—which you may notice are also symptoms associated with depression and anxiety.

We depend on our guts to help us properly digest and absorb the food we consume each day. Without the gut, we couldn't get the nutrients we need to survive, let alone thrive. But it's much more than just a consumptive organ. The gut also happens to be the largest endocrine, or hormone-secreting, organ in mammals—and, as such, plays a pivotal role in the immune response. It helps mediate when, where, and how pro-inflammatory molecules are deployed in the body and brain. It's also home to hundreds of neurons, believe it or not: the largest number of neurons outside the brain.

All in all, the GI tract is a pretty amazing organ. It incessantly chats back and forth with our brains. That said, it doesn't work alone, but instead relies on the microbiome—trillions of microorganisms, including bacteria, archaea, fungi, viruses, and other parasites that live within the GI tract—to help it transfer the right information to the brain for optimal functioning. This new understanding of how our gut and mind interact marks an exciting new area in both depression and anxiety research by providing more evidence that diet can help us to better manage our mental health. After all, nothing affects the microbiome like what you eat.

MICROBIOME MEDIATION

As we discussed in the last chapter, inflammation is a major contributor to both depression and anxiety. Cryan put it nicely when he said once you understand that the immune system is involved in everything happening in your body, including your brain, and that the microbiome plays a large role in regulating the immune system, it becomes clear that the microbiome must be involved with mediating our brain health.

"It's incredibly complex. The microbiome is not a single entity, even though we talk about it as if it is a single thing," he said. "Rather, it is a sophisticated ecosystem of trillions of different microorganisms. You're dealing with a sort of rain forest effect here—and we are now learning this rain forest is producing all kinds of wonderful chemicals that support brain health in different ways."

It's a bit of a paradigm shift to think of microorganisms, particularly bacteria, as promoting health. Traditionally, we've thought of bacteria as harmful, disease-causing agents, but not all bacteria are pathogenic. Many of those we consider disease-causing, like *E. coli*, naturally live in the gut. It's only when we pick up particular variants, or their numbers grow too high inside our bodies, that we get sick. Most bacteria are silent, hidden passengers that travel along with us during our life's journey. It's a symbiotic relationship. They want us to stay healthy so they can grow and thrive, too. They need us as much as we need them.

Each and every one of us is born with a microbiome made up of the bacteria passed to you in utero and at birth by your mother. After birth, you then pick up new microbiome passengers as you breathe in the air, try new foods (as well as eat your old favorites), hug loved ones, explore outside, shake hands with strangers, or even cuddle with your cat or dog. Every single interaction with your environment has the power to change your microbiome—some subtly, some to a greater extent.

To stay healthy, you want a diverse microbiome, with a variety of good bugs, or what some call probiotics. Certainly, such good bugs help break down foods and synthesize vital nutrients, like B vitamins. They also produce the nourishment for the cells that line our gut by making short-chained fatty acids and modulate our inflammatory system. Without them, our bodies wouldn't achieve full nourishment; many nutrients would just pass on through us, and others wouldn't be produced at all. You can see why we rely on our microbiomes to help us get the most out of the foods we eat.

The microbiome also helps the gut send important messages to the brain. This goes beyond just letting your brain know you ate something questionable that should be purged as soon as possible. It's much more complex than that. You may wonder how scientists figured this out. It started with a study of germ-free animals. Germ-free mice or rats are pretty much exactly what they sound like—animals that are born and raised in sterile conditions so they can grow and develop without a microbiome. In fact, they don't

THE MICROBIOME

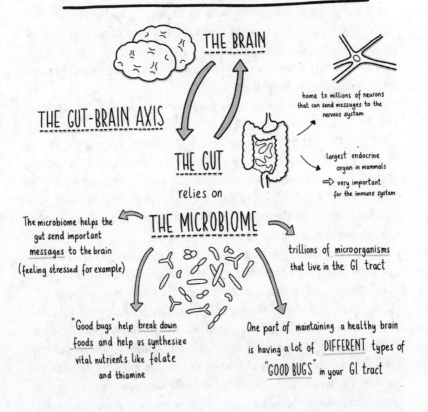

THE BRAIN

THE GUT-BRAIN AXIS

THE GUT

relies on

home to millions of neurons that can send messages to the nervous system

largest endocrine organ in mammals

⇨ very important for the immune system

The microbiome helps the gut send important messages to the brain
(feeling stressed for example)

THE MICROBIOME

trillions of microorganisms that live in the GI tract

"Good bugs" help break down foods and help us synthesize vital nutrients like folate and thiamine

One part of maintaining a healthy brain is having a lot of DIFFERENT types of "GOOD BUGS" in your GI tract

have any bacteria in or on their body at all. Researchers started using these special animals in the 1960s in nutrition studies, to better understand how bacteria helped us to digest and synthesize things like those important B vitamins. While these animals tend to exhibit slower growth, scientists, at the time, would have told you they were similar enough to typical animals—they just happened to be missing bacteria. But, as the years progressed, and the number of studies grew, scientists noticed some interesting behavioral differences. One of those was how germ-free animals responded to stress. They had a lot of trouble coping when the going got tough, like having to interact with new animals or moving to a strange habitat.

In 2004, researchers from Japan's Kyushu University decided to take a closer look at the brains of these germ-free mice to see why they were so susceptible to stress issues. They restrained both germ-free mice and normal mice using a small, conical tube for one hour. It's a tight fit in these tubes—and, as you can imagine, after sixty minutes of being unable to escape, let alone move all that much, the animals were not very happy. When the scientists looked at the stress response after this forced restraint, they found something really interesting—what they termed an "exaggerated" response to the stress.

Upon observing the animals, the scientists saw that the germ-free mice were much more freaked out by the experience, cowering in fear in their normal habitats for a long time after the restraint task had ended. They also showed physiological differences, too. Levels of specific hormones that are known to be released during stress, like cortisol, were substantially higher in the germ-free animals than the other mice. And when the scientists took a look at BDNF levels in the cortex and hippocampus of the germ-free brains, they saw expression of the brain-fertilizing neurotrophin was much lower in this group. Put it all together and the germ-free animals were at a distinct disadvantage when it came to managing this stressful situation as compared to mice who had an intact microbiome—and that disadvantage was linked to interesting changes in the brain.

That result, in and of itself, is pretty fascinating. But the Kyushu researchers took things one step further. They repeated the experiment after giving those germ-free mice a probiotic. When the scientists reconstituted their guts with *Bifidobacterium infantis*, a "friendly," good bug bacterium usually found in the microbiome that helps with digestion and vitamin synthesis, they reversed that out-of-control stress response. The formerly germ-free mice handled it as well as other mice, cowering for a bit after the restraint but then soon returning to normal mousey behavior.[1] These researchers showed that having the right bacteria in your GI tract could change the way your brain responded to stress. It's remarkable.

We see this link between the microbiome and serious mental illness in actual patients as well. Psychiatrists at Houston Methodist Hospital recently analyzed the microbiomes of 111 adult inpatients who had come to the hospital due to serious mental illness, such as severe depression or anxiety. They found that the less diverse the microbiome, the more serious a patient's psychiatric symptoms were. What's more, those patients with more diversity and richness in their gut bacteria were more likely to remit from their condition—and to do so more quickly.[2]

It's now quite clear that, when it comes to depression and anxiety, the microbiome matters—and matters greatly. If we can find ways to improve the microbiome, we may have another way to fight mental health issues.

BACTERIA AND THE STRESS RESPONSE

As striking as these studies may be, optimal brain health doesn't come down to one bacterial strain. There are literally trillions of different bugs inside your gut. And, like I said before, most of them, in the right amounts, aren't harmful at all. In fact, they can do amazing things for your overall health and well-being, from helping to digest your food to releasing those wonderful chemicals that Cryan talked about, thus providing key information that travels directly from your gut to your brain. We now understand that one part of maintaining a healthy mood is having a lot of different types of good bugs hanging out in your GI tract, a condition that is often referred to as microbiome diversity.

"About ten years ago, a variety of studies just came together—

about the microbiome and inflammation and that you need a microbiome for normal brain development and a healthy stress response," said Cryan. "The next step for us was to better understand how the microbiome might influence conditions like depression and anxiety and whether it could help us find ways to reverse it."

We've long known that early life stress, such as physical abuse or extreme poverty, can change your brain in ways that increase your likelihood of developing a mental health issue later in life. It also happens to change the diversity of your microbiome. Cryan's early research discovered that rats who had been significantly stressed early in life had reduced microbiome diversity in their guts. It's unclear whether this is because of the stress of poverty itself or the fresh fruits and vegetables that can help populate your gut with good bugs are less available in poorer communities. It's likely a combination of the two.

Given that fact, it's probably not a surprise to learn that when Cryan and his colleagues looked at depressed or anxious humans, they found reduced bacteria diversity in their GI tracts, too. While it's unclear whether a lack of certain types of bacteria may lead to depression or if depression somehow reduces those bacteria in the gut is unknown; it may well be a bit of both. But, Cryan said, this strong association offers the possibility that simply finding ways to get some of those good bugs back into the GI tract could help people better manage their depressive or anxious symptoms.[3]

Interestingly enough, problems like Susan's IBS are also more likely when you have reduced diversity in the microbiome, which may be one reason why we see so many gastrointestinal troubles traveling with depression and anxiety. Having too much of certain types of bacteria in the gut can lead to both physical illness and mental health symptoms. But those good bugs, or health-promoting strains of bacteria in the gut, can counter them. Animal studies strongly suggest higher concentrations of bacterial species like *lactobacillus* and *bifidobacterium* in the GI tract can help improve cognitive function and reduce an animal's reactivity to stress.

There are likely many more strains, currently unknown, that also contribute to brain health. And when Cryan and his colleagues held a small trial to test the addition of a single bacterium, *Bifidobacterium longum* 1714, to the diet of healthy volunteers, they found similar results.[4]

Cryan recruited a group of twenty-two male university students to participate in the study. He assessed their stress levels, depression and anxiety symptoms, and basic cognitive function. Measuring stress in people can be done in a variety of ways. You can give different questionnaires and ask them to report how they feel. You can also measure the body's response to stress. Some common ways to do this include measuring skin conductance; when you are stressed out or feeling emotional, you'll see more electrical activity in the skin, which reflects your body's arousal. You can also measure circulating levels of stress hormones, like cortisol. When a person shows increased skin conductance and higher levels of cortisol, it's pretty safe to say they're stressed out.

One of the tasks that Cryan and his associates had the study participants do is called the socially evaluated cold pressor task. It's not much fun. Basically, you need to submerge your nondominant hand into ice-cold water—39 degrees Fahrenheit—for a period of four minutes. Just having your arm in the water is a reliable stressor. Healthy people generally show quite increased elevated levels of cortisol after doing it, but the social evaluation really ups the ante.

"While your arm is submerged, someone's watching, taking notes, and maybe even making comments on how you are doing," he said. "It's really quite unpleasant."

After that initial testing session, half of the participants were then given sachets with *Bifidobacterium longum* 1714 to tip into their milk each morning. Controls were given a placebo. After a month, Cryan and colleagues reassessed the students by performing the same evaluations, including the socially evaluated cold pressor task. They then switched things up. This time, they gave the people who were initially in the control group sachets of the probiotics to take for the next month while the others received a placebo. Four weeks later, everyone came back to the lab and did it all again. When Cryan examined the data, he found the study participants who were taking the probiotic reported feeling less anxious, had less of a physiological stress response to the cold pressor task, and even showed some enhanced memory skills.

"It was a small study, but the results were really encouraging," said Cryan. "We saw the probiotic reduced both how they reported their stress levels and the physiology of their stress response in the body. If we could see similar improvements in a person in even a mildly depressed or anxious situation, it could make a huge difference."

The results, in fact, were so encouraging that Paul Enck, a researcher at the University of Tübingen in Germany, wanted to see what kind of brain activity might be mediating these stress-reducing effects. Instead of cold water, he used a computer game to induce stress. It's called Cyberball, and is simply a pong-like game where you virtually pass a ball between yourself and two others. There are two conditions in this game: the first is inclusion that you and your two partners play by passing the ball back and forth in a friendly manner; the second, the exclusion condition, means that, at some point, this friendly game of catch will turn into "Monkey in the Middle"—and you, unfortunately, get to play the role of the monkey. The other two virtual players will play on and not throw you the ball no matter what you do. It's another task that can reliably bring on a strong stress response.

"It takes you back to childhood and feeling like you've been excluded from the social group," said Cryan. "The task is quite well-validated—and it shows us the brain really doesn't like this sort of social distress."

Enck and colleagues recruited forty healthy volunteers to take *Bifidobacterium longum* 1714 or a placebo for four weeks. They then invited them back to the lab to have their brain activity and stress response measured while playing Cyberball. Afterward, participants were asked to fill out questionnaires about the experience. They found that the volunteers who took the probiotic not only showed a smaller stress response to the exclusion condition of the game, but they also showed changes in brain activity. Those changes, the authors argued, were indicative of "enhanced vitality and reduced mental fatigue."[5]

Bifidobacterium longum 1714 is certainly not the only good bug that can improve stress, mood, or anxiety symptoms in healthy individuals. Several other studies have shown that a few different strains can offer the same benefits. Taken together, what we see is that these good bugs seem to help the brain be a little more resilient in the face of stress. And, in doing so, they support the idea that you need a healthy gut—and a diverse microbiome—to have a healthy brain.

HOW, EXACTLY, DO GOOD BUGS WORK ON THE BRAIN?

How might these tiny bacteria manage such impressive effects? We already talked at length about how inflammation can affect the brain. Higher concentrations of unhealthy bugs can summon pro-inflammatory responses that dampen activity in well-established learning, memory, reward-processing, and emotional circuits in the brain. I also mentioned those hundreds of millions of neurons in the gut. As it so happens, the majority of serotonin neurons—the neurons that release the neurotransmitter that help regulate mood and learning—are located in the gut, not the brain.

These serotonin-releasing neurons can be activated by rare and unique cells that line the intestines called enterochromaffin cells. The enterochromaffin cells act as sensors, detecting the different peptides, or short chains of amino acids, released by different members of the microbiome. They then tell those serotonin neurons where, when, and how much of the neurotransmitter to release into the nervous system.[6] The levels of serotonin in the nervous system can then go on to influence the release of other vital neurotransmitters like glutamate and dopamine where needed. When gut microbe diversity is compromised, the second-order effects to brain systems that help regulate mental health can be quite dire.[7]

There's also a third mode of communication through one of the body's cranial nerves called the vagus nerve. The vagus nerve has its fingers in almost all of the bodily organs. It's been shown to have strong involvement in both modulating hunger and stress and regulating the immune response, including mediating inflammation, via its nerve fibers. When the vagus nerve is electrically stimulated, as it was in the past to treat stubborn forms of epilepsy, one of the side effects was an improvement in mood. Interestingly enough, this sort of stimulation is also sometimes used today to help with treatment-resistant depression. A vagus nerve stimulation device was even approved by the Food and Drug Administration as a treatment in 2005.

Think of the vagus nerve like a switchboard operator. It passes all kinds of messages back and forth between the viscera and the brain. New studies now show that gut bacteria can pass messages to the vagus nerve via hormones, like the cortisol released after stress; the nutrients you eat from food; and the peptides made and released by the bacteria themselves. Those messages can then be passed on to the nervous system within milliseconds, thanks to the vagus being so well-connected. For example, *Lactobacillus rhamnosus*, a good bug that has been linked to improving anxiety symptoms, works its magic by talking to the vagus nerve. When this nerve is cut, those effects are completely gone.[8]

It's pretty complicated. There's a lot of information zooming back and forth between the gut and the brain that helps keep us healthy, and scientists are only beginning to understand all the ways that the microbiome can affect brain function through the gut-brain axis. Yet, despite all the complexity, and the work that continues to be done to unravel it, what's become utterly clear is that a healthy gut is a prerequisite for a healthy brain.

PROBIOTICS AS A TREATMENT

As seen in the study at Houston Methodist Hospital, increased diversity in the gut can help with symptom improvement. What might happen when we give patients probiotic treatment? In the case of bipolar disorder, researchers at Johns Hopkins University followed sixty-six patients who were hospitalized after a severe manic episode. Half of those patients were given a probiotic supplement, which included *Lactobacillus rhamnosus* GG and *Bifidobacterium animalis*, to take for twenty-four weeks after discharge. During that twenty-four-week observation period, twenty-four of the thirty-three individuals in the placebo group were re-hospitalized—but only eight of those in the probiotic group returned to the hospital and, when they did return, required less in-patient treatment time. When the study authors looked at the patients' inflammation levels, they discovered that those who had abnormally high pro-inflammatory molecules in the body were most helped by the probiotics. The results suggest that probiotics can help dampen intestinal inflammation and, by doing so, modulate the symptoms associated with bipolar disorder.

There have also been trials that show that regular supplementation with probiotics can lead to improvements in depression and anxiety symptoms. In a recent meta-analysis of existing clinical trials that used some probiotic strain as a treatment—studies use different bugs for different reasons—researchers from China's Central South University found they did have beneficial effects, reducing reported symptoms and distress related to depression.[9] Similar reviews have found that probiotics can also help relieve anxiety symptoms.[10] That said, because of the different strains and different amounts used, it's unclear what protocol works best. It should also be noted that several trials haven't shown positive results, which is why adding some random probiotic supplement to your breakfast each day may not be the best way to beat or treat your depression or anxiety.

As Cryan said, the microbiome is very complex. While you can give people a probiotic, you can't necessarily stop them from eating foods that may negate its effects. Many of the highly processed, sugary, fatty, prepackaged foods so common to the Western diet give more sustenance to the "bad bugs," or the bacterial strains that get in the way of positive mood. Those foods can also promote the release of pro-inflammatory molecules that negatively affect brain health.

It's also important to mention, Cryan added, that everyone's microbiome—thanks to their backgrounds and experiences—are different. One probiotic supplement might work for one person but have no effect on another. Some might need a higher dose of a probiotic to reduce depression or anxiety symptoms; some may need a mixture of different strains. There have even been some studies now showing that ingesting too much of even brain-healthy strains can cause problems like gas, bloating, and even brain fog. Figuring out the proper supplementation doses for each individual is tricky. That's why, he said, one of the best ways to influence the mind through the microbiome is through making changes to your diet. It not only can help to populate those good bugs, it can provide the important fiber content that the healthy bacteria that are already living in your gut can thrive upon.

"If you could modify diet to increase levels of certain bacterial species that we know can help the brain, that could be beneficial," he said. He is currently running a study to look at the effect of adding foods that we know to help feed good bugs, like fermented foods and fiber, to see whether it has any effect on mood.

While Cryan's full results are not available yet, he recently shared some preliminary findings on the popular BBC television show *Trust Me, I'm a Doctor*. He recruited eight healthy volunteers to participate: half continued eating as they regularly do and the other half were put on what Cryan calls a "psychobiotic" diet, or one full of fermented foods like kefir, sauerkraut, and probiotic yogurt, as well as fiber-rich foods that have been shown to feed healthy bacteria in the gut, including onions and berries. When Cryan and colleagues assessed volunteers after a month, they found that those on the psychobiotic diet had developed a more diverse microbiome as well as a reduced physiological response to stress.

"Even short term, we could shift the microbiome and the ability to deal with stress," he said. "It's a very small study but even seeing these results in such a small group is heartening. We plan to continue with a much larger group of people so we can really look at this."

These results, preliminary though they are, fit well with the dietary intervention studies published by Felice Jacka and others. Following a plant-based diet, like the Mediterranean diet, with the addition of fermented foods, can help promote a healthy gut by increasing the number of good bugs, like *lactobacillus* and *bifidobacteria*, in the microbiome. Furthermore, upping the amount of fiber in your diet with the consumption of whole fruits and vegetables will not only help keep you more regular and keep any gut issues at bay, it can also give those good bugs the food they need to thrive. As a bonus, in making such changes to your diet, you can lower inflammation, increase the release of serotonin, and promote overall brain health.

Susan, though skeptical at first, started to feel much better as she found ways to add more fermented foods and fiber to her diet. Not only did it help her with her worries and improve her sleep, it also gave her remarkable relief from her IBS symptoms. The addition of daily kefir in her morning smoothies, as well as more legumes in her go-to salads, made a big difference in the way she felt and how she responded to stress.

"I feel a big difference in both my belly and my brain when I don't get enough of these foods," she said. "Sometimes, I'm just not paying attention. Things get so busy that I'm just eating whatever's

Nutrients for Brain Health:

FIBER

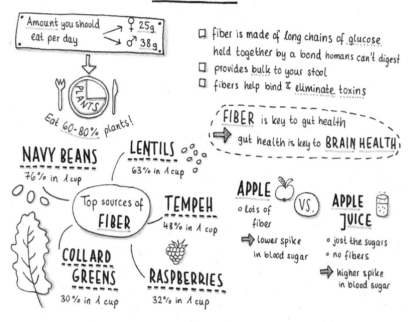

- Amount you should eat per day → ♀ 25g → ♂ 38g

Eat 60–80% plants!

☐ fiber is made of long chains of glucose held together by a bond humans can't digest
☐ provides bulk to your stool
☐ fibers help bind & eliminate toxins

FIBER is key to gut health
→ gut health is key to BRAIN HEALTH

NAVY BEANS
76% in 1 cup

LENTILS
63% in 1 cup

Top sources of **FIBER**

TEMPEH
48% in 1 cup

COLLARD GREENS
30% in 1 cup

RASPBERRIES
32% in 1 cup

APPLE
∘ lots of fiber
→ lower spike in blood sugar

VS.

APPLE JUICE
∘ just the sugars
∘ no fibers
→ higher spike in blood sugar

around. But within a day or two, I can feel it. I'm like, 'Time to get my good bugs back in order.'"

Take a good look at your plate during your next meal. Are you eating in a way to benefit your microbiome? Are you including fermented foods to increase the amount of good bugs that live there? Are you eating mainly plants, including high-fiber foods that can feed those gut bacteria—and, consequently, your brain?

What you should be looking for is a plate full of fiber, from your favorite greens, veggies, beans, nuts, and whole grains. Yogurt, kefir, and sauerkraut and other fermented foods are also great sources of good bugs. If your plate is lacking these items, maybe it's time to start adding them in, slowly but surely. It's both an established way to eat to beat depression and anxiety and one of the key elements of the Eat to Beat Depression and Anxiety Six-Week Plan that will put all of this knowledge and science to work for you.

CHAPTER 4: Recap

- The microbiome, the trillions of microorganisms, including bacteria, fungi, viruses, and parasites that live within the GI tract, also help to mediate mental health in a variety of ways.

- Each and every one of us is born with a microbiome made up of the bacteria passed to us in utero and during birth by our mothers. After birth, you then pick up new microbiome passengers as you breathe in the air, try new foods (as well as eat your old favorites), hug loved ones, explore outside, or even cuddle with your cat or dog. Every single interaction with your environment has the power to change your microbiome—some subtly, others to a greater extent. To stay healthy, you want a diverse microbiome, with a variety of good bugs, also known as probiotics.

- Those good bugs not only help us digest our food but also send important messages to the brain. When you don't have these important bacteria in the gut, brain function—and mental health—suffer. There is a strong correlation between reduced diversity in the microbiome and both depression and anxiety.

- Research studies have shown that the addition of specific strains of bacteria to the microbiome can help both animals and human beings change the way the brain responds to stress, making it more resilient.

- While some might look at this work as a sign to take a probiotic supplement—and some studies have shown improvement in depressive and anxiety symptoms in doing so—one of the easiest ways to up the diversity in your own microbiome is to eat foods that promote good bugs. This includes fiber, from veggies, to feed those bugs, as well as fermented foods to repopulate different strains of healthy bacteria directly to your gut.

· · · · · · ·

Chapter 5

THE BEST FOODS TO BEAT DEPRESSION AND ANXIETY

From *Fifty Shades of Kale* to Reformed Kale Evangelist

I have a confession to make: I'm a reformed kale evangelist.

Those of you who know me and have followed my work over the past decade know that I'm a big fan of kale. It's probably fair to say that I adore this particular plant—I even wrote a cookbook about it called *Fifty Shades of Kale*. Simply put, I consider it my spirit vegetable.

It might be hard for some to understand how I developed such an affinity for this leafy green. About twelve years ago, my wife, Lucy, and I moved to an apartment in New York's West Village neighborhood. After spending so much time away from my family's farm, this Indiana boy was missing wide-open spaces and fresh food. Luckily, just steps from our new front door was the Abingdon Square Greenmarket, a weekly farmers market that brought local farmers, fishmongers, and butchers to the tiny park at the intersection of Hudson and West 12th Streets. I started spending my Saturday mornings there, picking up our food for the week. Suddenly, my diet was filled with seasonal farm-fresh options again. And the farmers, known for their neighborliness, were happy to spend time talking to me about the produce they had to offer as well as our shared experience of living on a farm. I felt like I was a part of something—this amazing market gave me a new way to connect the city and country parts of myself.

One of the farmers I befriended at the Greenmarket was named Dave Siegel. He and his partner Jessica Swadosh had a five-acre spread in upstate New York called Muddy Farm. Each week, Farmer Dave and Farmer Jess brought in gorgeous produce for the market goers. Their offerings included five different varieties of kale: lacinato, green curly, red Russian, rainbow lacinato, and blue vates. Dave would artfully stack bunches of each on a table under a tent and we'd talk about their unique properties. At the time, kale was just starting to pop up on the menus of popular restaurants around the city. I started trying as many varietals as we could.

Coincidentally, this was also the time I started realizing how little I knew about how food impacts mental health. As a psychiatrist, I needed that to change. The Food as Medicine movement was taking hold, and the more I learned, the more I realized that physicians like me needed to do more to help our patients get the nutrients their bodies were craving. Kale is incredibly nutrient dense, each bite packed with vital vitamins and minerals. With so many amazing cultivars on Farmer Dave's table, kale seemed to me like a food that could help both my family and my patients get more of those nutrients and help their brains in the process.

Of course, it didn't hurt that I also really enjoyed eating this vegetable. From the traditional sukuma wiki—a tasty mix of sautéed kale and collards—I got hooked on while working in the psychiatric ward of a Kenyan hospital as a medical student to the amazing salads now gracing the menus of the toniest bistros in New York, I couldn't get enough kale.

You'd think writing a book like *Fifty Shades of Kale* would get this green out of my system (I even planted fifty-four varieties of kale on our farm!). Yet, it was just the beginning of my kale mania.

My goal was to empower people to eat more greens, to find ways to make kale more palatable so more people could easily incorporate it into a healthy diet. We even launched National Kale Day, on the first Wednesday of every October, to help raise awareness of this leafy green's powerful nutrient punch. There were kale parties, kale T-shirts, kale stickers, and even kale cocktails. We helped schools and hospitals around the country start serving kale and even partnered with the Department of Defense on Operation Kale and stocked every commissary in the United States. It was my effort at promoting a national brain health intervention using food.

Then, over time, I noticed something troubling. I still loved kale with a passion and tried to educate people about why it was such a great brain-boosting food. But as I traveled around the country, giving talks and going to different events, more and more people would tell me, usually whispered with some embarrassment, that they just didn't like kale. They might be forcing it down on occasion in order to eat healthier, but they did not enjoy it. A good friend of mine, who is also a physician, confided that he, too, despised my beloved green. He admitted, "It tastes like dirt and stones to me."

I noticed a similar trend in some of my patients. As we discussed their diets, and where they might make changes to help reduce depression and anxiety symptoms, I'd see a look of disgust on more than a few faces when I mentioned kale. I quickly realized that it didn't matter how much I educated people about this brain-nutrient power player, or even how well I might dress it up with amazing new recipes—some people just weren't going to go there.

I realized that obviously people weren't going to reap the nutritional benefits of kale if they couldn't stand the stuff. That was the start of my conversion to reformed kale evangelist. I still love this vegetable and want anyone with a brain to understand how remarkable it is from a nutrient-density standpoint. I'm still going to share every great kale recipe I come across and make homemade kale chips. But I now better appreciate that we all have different tastes—as well as some challenges—when it comes to food. Kale is a "superfood" for me, not just because of its nutrient count or even that I enjoy eating it. There's also a psychological component to my affection: kale gives me a taste of my farm roots even when I'm in the middle of the city. It makes me feel at home.

Now that I've made that connection, I understand that kale may not have the same appeal to you as it does to me. Your go-to green may be arugula or baby spinach. You may revel in romaine or go radical with radicchio. Maybe you're someone who appreciates a nice, crisp watercress. Whatever you enjoy the most is great—and that's the leafy green you should eat. So, while I'll continue to celebrate National Kale Day, the first Wednesday of October (and several times a week every month of the year), you don't have to. You can get the vital fiber, vitamin C, folate, phytonutrients, and other brain-healthy nutrients from the leafy veggie of your choice.

UNDERSTANDING FOOD CATEGORIES

We already talked about the twelve nutrients—plus a few more—that have been linked to both the prevention and management of depression and anxiety. While it's important, from a scientific standpoint, to highlight those nutrients, talking about vitamins and minerals doesn't do much to change people's diets. According to the Centers for Disease Control and Prevention, deficiencies in nutrients including iron, vitamin A, and zinc remain a serious issue—with more than two billion people across the globe suffering from some sort of micronutrient deficiency. Telling people to up their vitamin B12 can only take you so far—and, generally, it tends to inspire people to hit the supermarket supplement aisle instead of eating a more balanced diet. That's not our goal here.

When we try to think beyond nutrients, too often conversations turn to one "superfood" or another. For example, you've likely heard experts talk about the health properties of blueberries, green tea, wild salmon, and broccoli sprouts. I'll admit I'm guilty of this with my kale advocacy work—hence, my reformed status. Again, these are all great foods. They are all chock-full of healthy nutrients that promote brain health and are a great addition to any diet. But eating to beat depression and anxiety requires you to think beyond just adding a superfood or two to your menu planning. To help the brain work its best, I've learned, it's more valuable to think more broadly about your diet in terms of food *categories.*

Food categories are exactly what they sound like—groupings of foods that contain high levels of brain-healthy nutrients. When Dr. LaChance and I created the AFS and started to make food recommendations based on the nutrients contained within it, we quickly realized that many of these essential nutrients travel together. Kale is rich in antidepressant and anti-anxiety vitamins, minerals, phytonutrients, and fiber. But so are Swiss chard and arugula. Pumpkin seeds are a great vehicle to get fiber and zinc. But walnuts, oysters, and chickpeas also pack a nutritional punch. Let the experts fight about whether broccoli is nutritionally superior to kale—or if brussels sprouts have them both beat in the vitamin K department. Ultimately, whether one has more of a certain phytonutrient than the other is a moot point if people aren't willing to eat these foods in the first place. And as we discussed, too often, they aren't.

As I talked to more people, including my patients, about their likes and dislikes regarding food, it became clear that focusing on these broader categories made it easier for them to consider making small changes that could have a big impact on their symptoms. It also made it easier to keep track of the changes they did make—and where they could make further improvements. When it comes to food, like most health interventions, you need to find ways to meet people where they are.

As a psychiatrist who now understands the impact of food choices on mental health, I speak with each of my patients in detail about what they eat. When I introduce the concept of food categories, invariably, I'll hear "I don't like that" about one food or another. For example, when Pete first came to see me, he was adamant that he didn't like seafood, one of our top categories for beating depression and anxiety. I'll be honest, I didn't blame him. I didn't always like it much, either. It took a lot of experimentation to find seafood that I enjoyed—and I told him as much. But as we talked more about his aversion to it, I quickly learned that the only fish he had ever really eaten was a mushy, tasteless sole that his grandmother served during the holidays when he was a kid. He had never tried mussels, shrimp, or salmon. He hadn't experienced good sushi, either. At some point, he had decided seafood wasn't for him and found himself stuck in that mind-set.

To help open him up to the possibility that he might not hate all *fruits de mer*, I gave Pete some homework. I knew from our food discussions that he loved Mexican cuisine and frequently ordered takeout from a restaurant near his home. I asked him to put in an order for a fish taco that week and to try just a single bite. If he didn't like it, he could simply put it down and walk away. When I saw him the week after, he told me he was surprised at how good the mahi-mahi taco was.

"The spices were really good," Pete said. "It was hard for me to even tell it was fish and not chicken."

Since then, Pete has explored a number of different seafood options that he can easily add to his diet. Some, like sardines and sole, aren't foods he will ever enjoy anytime soon. They don't work for him: "too fishy." (I'm hopeful.) But other options in the seafood food category, like wild-caught mahi-mahi, shrimp, and salmon ended up being quite easy for him to add to his favorite tacos—and have become staples of his diet. As he said, when he doesn't eat right, he doesn't feel right. Making sure he eats seafood regularly helps him feel right.

By focusing on categories over food—like "seafood" over "sole"—you have the opportunity to make a swap here, add a new food there, or make a small change in any part of your diet. It's a message we all need to remember sometimes: to eat to beat depression and anxiety, make small changes and keep exploring as an eater.

THE TOP FOOD CATEGORIES TO BEAT
DEPRESSION AND ANXIETY

People who've been diagnosed with anxiety or depression often experience decreased motivation and a lack of joy. Trying to convince them to take on a dietary pattern with a fixed—and often complex—menu plan is often too daunting. Frankly, it's discouraging. However, as I said in the beginning, this is a book for eaters. And eaters know that food can be one of life's greatest joys; it shouldn't be just another thing you have to endure.

Our relationships with food can be complex. There are the foods we love to savor—and the foods that we gulp down in a rush. There are foods we automatically go to when we're feeling down or in need of comfort. There may be others that we favor when we're sharing with our friends and loved ones. And, of course, there are foods that we won't touch with a ten-foot pole. Each one of us has unique tastes and strong values surrounding what we eat. Those tastes and values are as individual as your experiences with depression and anxiety. That's why it should be entirely up to you to pick the foods you enjoy most from each food category. That said, for each category, I will suggest the "power players"—foods in the grouping that are both particularly nutrient dense and easy to add to some of your favorite dishes, just in case you're looking for a place to start.

I want to emphasize that each and every one of us approaches food from different perspectives. Some of us are strictly vegan. Others are walking the keto path. Certain people need to honor specific food allergies or sensitivities as they consider making dietary changes. I'm meeting more and more people who are trying to limit their sugar intake. We all have our own needs and desires when it comes to the foods we eat. That's another benefit of using food categories instead of specific foods. If a certain item, or even a certain category as a whole, doesn't work with the way you like to eat, there's always an alternative to help you get the nutrients you need. The recommended power players are only a suggestion.

So, pick the foods you enjoy eating. That's one reason there are smoothie, pesto, and salad formulas later in this book—to enable you to easily substitute your favorite. Sub out kale for a green you have a deeper appreciation for in the pesto on page 185 or the smoothies on page 225. Eat it your way! The only essential ingredient besides unprocessed foods, from my perspective, is a certain amount of joyfulness that should come along with whatever you select.

There are a variety of food categories that can aid in your quest for a healthier brain—and remission from depression and anxiety symptoms. They are leafy greens; rainbow fruits and veggies; seafood; nuts, beans, and seeds; meat; eggs and dairy; fermented foods; and dark chocolate. Foods from these groups contain the important nutrients you need to feed the good bugs in your gut, reduce inflammation, and put your brain into "grow mode." All things that can help with depression and anxiety.

Leafy Greens (and Other Colors, Too)

Whether they are green, purple, or some other color, leafy vegetables give you the most bang for your buck when you're talking about nutrient density, the nutrient-to-calorie ratio. Spinach, kale, watercress, arugula, collards, beet greens, and chard are all great for getting your daily dose of fiber, vitamin C, vitamin A, and folate. And, thanks to the bright colors in the leaves, they're full of healthy phytonutrients, too. Eating more leaves means you are getting more hydration, satiation, and nutrient density in every meal.

But one of the best things about leafy veggies is their culinary versatility. You can enjoy these foods in salads, soups, or stir-fries. You can blend them up into a tasty pesto to throw on chicken or over pasta. Add them to smoothies or even muffins. There's really no limit to what you can do. Furthermore, the price point for a bunch of greens is pretty low—usually just a few bucks—and they can last in the fridge for a good while. Leafy vegetables are a great staple to have around to use as the foundation for a variety of brain-boosting meals.

I've included seaweed in this section, though technically it is an alga. These leafy greens of the sea are the most concentrated source of iodine, a nutrient that didn't make our list but is essential for brain health as thyroid function depends on iodine. Iodine levels in the United States have long been in decline, and having low iodine during pregnancy is a top cause of development delay in children worldwide. As if that's not reason enough, seaweed is also an excellent source of fiber, iron, zinc, and phytonutrients.

Power players: *Kale and seaweed*

Recommended consumption: *2 to 3 cups of leafy greens per day, 1 small serving of seaweed per week*

Rainbow Fruits and Vegetables

Take a good look at your plate. Is it full of color? Or do you see mostly beiges and browns? If you answered the latter, it's time to rethink.

Eating rainbow fruits and vegetables, like tomatoes, avocados, bell peppers, broccoli, cauliflower, and berries, is a great way to not only get important phytonutrients called flavonoids and carotenoids, but also fiber for the good bugs in your gut to thrive on. Flavonoids are responsible for the bright colors of these foods—and you can only get these health-promoting molecules in the plants you eat. Purple foods have anthocyanins. Orange gives you carotenoids. Reds signal lycopene. And all of them have powerful antioxidant and DNA-enhancing properties and can help keep pro-inflammatory molecules at bay—and, in the process, help keep your brain fighting fit.

That said, I want to give a special shout-out to anthocyanins, the compounds you can find in reddish-purplish foods ranging from blackberries to red cabbage. I don't like to play favorites, but these molecules are something special. These flavonoids have long been known to exhibit extraordinary anti-inflammatory properties. That's not much of a surprise. They have also been linked to improved memory and mood states. But scientists from the Centre for Research in Health Technologies and Information Systems in Porto, Portugal, recently discovered the way they do the voodoo they do so well is mediated through the microbiome.[1]

When you eat that bowl of blueberries or tuck into a great piece of eggplant Parmesan, those anthocyanins tell the body to produce more of a neuroprotective molecule called kynurenic acid through special messages they send the brain through the microbiome. This molecule has the power to facilitate sleep, boost mood, and decrease feelings of brain fog. And, of course, to help reduce inflammation in both the gut and the brain. These are all things, as you now know, that can help you in your fight against depression and anxiety.

Another tool to help you is the avocado. This is a special food—a favorite of brain health advocates, due to its high fat and phytonutrient content. These fruits are 82 percent fat, mostly monounsaturated fats. That's rare in the plant world. These fats help with the absorption of other phytonutrients, like lycopene, and that's one reason it is a power player for this food category, it boosts the effect of your eating rainbows. Another reason it is great for your plate is it's high content of fiber, potassium, and vitamin E, which didn't make the AFS list of nutrients, but is clearly linked to depression and improved brain health. Protect your special brain fat, eat more avocados.

Your greens and rainbows should be major constituents of your meals. Luckily, like greens, rainbows are also very versatile. You can use berries to counter the bitterness of certain greens or to sweeten up kefir or yogurt. Veggies like tomatoes and peppers are easily roasted, stir-fried, or used as the basis of pasta sauces and stews. You can dip your favorite raw veggies into hummus (page 219), guacamole, or ranch dip. And you can't go wrong snacking on your favorite berries and fruits. There are so many ways to eat the rainbow. You just need to find the way that works best for you.

Power players: *Red peppers and avocados*

Recommended consumption: *A mix of rainbow plants, at least 2 to 3 cups per day*

Seafood

This is often the most challenging food category for people to take on. As I admitted earlier, it certainly was for me. It took some time to try new things and figure out what kinds of seafood I actually enjoyed. Even those who typically turn their nose up at fish can often find ways to successfully add seafood into their diets. It's a great strategy to get those long-chain omega-3 fatty acids that your brain so desperately needs. Sardines, oysters, mussels, salmon, and cod are also chock-full of B12, selenium, iron, zinc, and protein.

A lot of people have concerns about fish, especially around mercury and microplastics. But this food group can truly make a huge difference when it comes to preventing and managing depression and anxiety symptoms. I strongly encourage you to avoid mercury and be aware of environmental toxins. One simple step is too simply to eat small fish and bivalves. With so many seasonings, sauces, and methods to prepare seafood, there's bound to be an option that will work for you and your brain. We'll focus more on seafood during the Eat to Beat Depression and Anxiety Six-Week Plan.

Power players: *Wild salmon, anchovies, and mussels*

Recommended consumption: *2 to 4 servings per week*

Nuts, Beans, and Seeds

This food category is regrettably often overlooked in the fight to beat depression and anxiety. From cashews to pumpkin seeds to lentils, nuts, seeds, and legumes are the top sources of plant-based protein. They're also rich in fiber, zinc, iron, and other essential vitamins. A relatively small serving offers a nice mix of healthy fats, protein, and slow-burning carbohydrates.

One of my favorite things about nuts, seeds, and legumes is that they make great snacks. When working with patients, one of the first things I suggest is replacing their current go-to snack food with some almonds, walnuts, and cashews. (Remember the study by Heather Francis we discussed earlier that gave nuts and nut butters to college students with depression?) Just a handful goes a long way as a midafternoon pick-me-up—helping your brain get the nutrients it needs and an extra boost of brain-derived neurotrophic factor (BDNF), the brain fertilizer we discussed in Chapter 3.

Beyond snacking, it's simple to add nuts, beans, and seeds to many of the dishes you're already eating and enjoying. It's easy to add some walnuts into a morning smoothie or to toss some pumpkin seeds on your favorite salad. Cashews are wonderful in a stir-fry. And don't forget beans. Throw a handful of black or red beans into your favorite soups or stews. (We even put beans in the Kefir Berry Smoothie on page 225.) These are all great options that can help you consume the nutrients you need to build a better brain.

Power players: *Pepitas (pumpkin seeds) and cashews; red beans*
Recommended consumption: *At least ¹/₂ to 1 cup of nuts and/or beans, and 1 tablespoon of seeds per day*

Meat

As a former vegetarian, I understand that many of us feel conflicted about eating meat. Some people won't ever do so—and that's fine. But, that said, meat is a remarkable source of iron, protein, and vitamin B12. As such, I've come to believe the age-old debate over whether we should or shouldn't eat meat instead needs to evolve into a discussion about how we can eat meat in a way that is both healthy for our bodies and sustainable for the environment. Foods like grass-fed beef, lamb, goat, and chicken can provide amazing flavors to our favorite dishes, as well as some important brain-boosting nutrients. Many small farms now focus on soil health and raising animals on pasture and grass, not feedlots. Finding your local farms and farmers is something I believe helps our mental health, and we'll talk more about this as part of the six-week plan.

Animals raised this way are better for the environment and produce healthier meat. Grass-fed beef has a third fewer calories than the meat that comes from grain-fed cows. It also boasts a different fatty acid profile—grass-fed beef has fewer omega-6 fatty acids, which helps to make sure your omega-3s are in balance and can do their job reducing inflammation and promoting brain health. But what grass-fed beef lacks in calories, it makes up for in nutrients. Because the animals freely roam and eat natural vegetation, you'll find more healthy fats, vitamin E, and carotenoids, as well as key vitamins and minerals, that your body and brain need to stay in tip-top shape. Liver is likely not a regular feature on your menu and may be one of the more challenging power players for many eaters. Still, ounce for ounce, liver is the most nutrient-dense part of an animal when it comes to brain nutrients such as B12, vitamin A, iron, and folate. Maybe this is one reason why our grandparents liked to eat pâté, add liver to ground beef and sausage, and enjoy a meal of chicken livers.

Power players: *Grass-fed beef and liver*
Recommended consumption: *3 servings per week*

Eggs and Dairy

Over the last few decades, eggs and dairy have seen more than their fair share of controversy in the nutrition world. But the egg, like kale, is an incredibly nutrient-dense food. A single egg is only 70 calories. Yet, this incredibly affordable and simple food also boasts an ideal complete protein, B vitamins, and choline, a cousin to the

B vitamins that has been linked to lower rates of anxiety symptoms. Eggs are also very easy to prepare and eat. Whether you boil one for a high-protein afternoon snack or whip up a rainbow vegetable frittata for your breakfast, eggs are an easy addition to your go-to meals.

My opinion of eggs is biased; we keep chickens on our farm. While writing this book, we incubated and hatched chicks from our own hens and rooster. Our chickens supply a near-continuous source of high-quality protein, B vitamins, and really everything to make a brain cell. Along with eggs, they provide nitrogen to fertilize the soil. All to say, eggs make sense to me as a farmer and a doctor.

Dairy, particularly fermented varieties like yogurt or kefir, can also be a welcome addition to your diet. These foods are full of the good bugs your body needs, as well as calcium and protein. However, like gluten, dairy has come under scrutiny in relation to inflammation. That may be because many of the most popular dairy items on grocery shelves, the reduced-fat milks and sweet yogurts, are highly processed and loaded with surprising amounts of sugar. It's also a food group that some people don't tolerate well. A few years ago I was forced to largely eliminate it from my diet, and today I have no issues with it.

However, even with the anti-dairy trend and my own experience, I still believe there are many interesting and healthy options from a variety of ruminants (sheep, cows, goats). We should remember dairy products are a consistent part of diets throughout the Mediterranean. Dairy isn't required eating, but certainly can be part of eating for better mental health and, like meat, a food category that's worthy of exploration.

Power players: *Eggs and fermented dairy, like unsweetened yogurt or kefir*

Recommended consumption: *5 to 7 eggs per week; 3 to 5 servings of dairy (ideally fermented) per week*

MEAT, EGGS & DAIRY

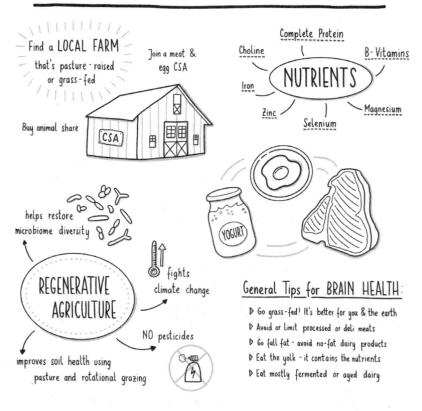

Find a LOCAL FARM
that's pasture-raised
or grass-fed

Join a meat &
egg CSA

Buy animal share

CSA

helps restore
microbiome diversity

REGENERATIVE
AGRICULTURE

fights
climate change

NO pesticides

improves soil health using
pasture and rotational grazing

Complete Protein

Choline   NUTRIENTS   B-Vitamins

Iron

Zinc   Selenium   Magnesium

YOGURT

General Tips for BRAIN HEALTH:

▷ Go grass-fed! It's better for you & the earth
▷ Avoid or limit processed or deli meats
▷ Go full fat - avoid no-fat dairy products
▷ Eat the yolk - it contains the nutrients
▷ Eat mostly fermented or aged dairy

Good Microbiome Bugs

This food category overlaps with many of the others above. In some
ways, that's not a surprise. In order to keep up maximum diversity
in your microbiome, you need to eat a variety of different foods.
The fiber from your rainbow veggies and beans will give all those
good bugs living in your gut the sustenance they need in order

to thrive. And regular consumption of fermented foods like kefir, yogurt, sauerkraut, miso, sourdough, kimchi, and kombucha will easily add more beneficial bacteria to your system to help support brain health.

Power players: *Kefir, miso, sauerkraut*

Recommended consumption: *3 to 5 servings of fermented foods per week*

Dark Chocolate

This final food category is, hands down, my favorite. Not only is it delicious but the specific flavanols contained within this treat—including epicatechin, a molecule shown to have wide-ranging cardiovascular benefits—are mighty good for your brain, too. People who eat higher amounts of dark chocolate have a 70 percent reduced risk of clinically relevant depression symptoms according to a study of 13,626 adults in the National Health and Examination Survey (NHANES). This benefit was not seen in those who consume milk chocolate.[2]

One of my colleagues, Scott A. Small, MD, a neurologist who heads the Alzheimer's Disease Research Center at Columbia University, made headlines in 2014 after showing that drinking a dark-chocolate beverage high in cocoa flavanols could improve memory function in older adults. Small and colleagues recruited thirty-seven individuals, between the ages of fifty and sixty-nine, to drink a cocoa beverage each day over a period of three months. Tough sell, right? About half of those individuals were given a beverage high in flavanols. The others were given one with a lower dose of these healthy molecules.

After the three-month period was over, Small and colleagues gave the study participants a memory test. Lo and behold, individuals who had consumed the higher flavanol beverage showed a 25 percent greater advantage on the memory task than those who didn't.[3] The researchers also showed it enhanced function of an area of the brain called the dentate gyrus, long associated with memory.

DARK CHOCOLATE

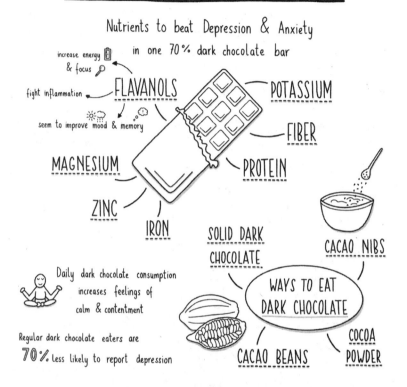

Nutrients to beat Depression & Anxiety in one 70% dark chocolate bar

increase energy & focus

FLAVANOLS

fight inflammation

seem to improve mood & memory

POTASSIUM

FIBER

MAGNESIUM

PROTEIN

ZINC

IRON

SOLID DARK CHOCOLATE

CACAO NIBS

Daily dark chocolate consumption increases feelings of calm & contentment

WAYS TO EAT DARK CHOCOLATE

Regular dark chocolate eaters are 70% less likely to report depression

CACAO BEANS

COCOA POWDER

You may ask what a memory test has to do with depression and anxiety. I'm glad you asked. Problems with thinking, poor concentration, and challenges with memory can be symptoms of depression and anxiety, too. Some hypothesize that flavanols like epicatechin work by suppressing inflammation—something we know also has benefits for mood. In addition, other studies have now demonstrated that 25 grams a day of polyphenol-rich dark chocolate can reduce salivary cortisol, a marker of both stress and anxiety and an individual's perception of stress.[4] Put it all together and you can see that regular consumption of dark chocolate has numerous brain benefits—and can help combat the brain fog, low mood, and stressful feelings that many people with depression or anxiety commonly experience. I highly recommend you go straight to the source and stock your cupboard with cacao beans and nibs, as well as a high quality cocoa powder. Look for dark chocolate with two ingredients, cacao and sugar, and a cacao content of at least 70 percent. The higher the percentage of cacao, the better it is for your brain. If people question your motives, let them know it is doctor recommended.

Power players: *Dark chocolate and cacao*

Recommended consumption: *Cacao beans or nibs and/or dark chocolate, 3 to 5 three-ounce servings per week*

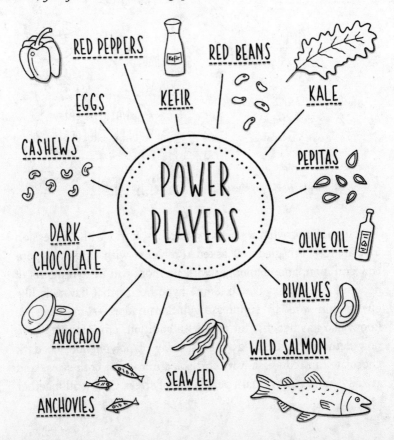

EATING TO BEAT DEPRESSION AND ANXIETY—YOUR WAY

Over the last few chapters, we've discussed the new science of Nutritional Psychiatry—and why the path to a stronger, more resilient brain begins at the end of your fork. You now know more about the nutrients that beat depression and anxiety, the foods that fight inflammation and promote brain growth, and the ways our microbiomes can affect our mental health. The foods you eat matter—and matter a great deal—when it comes to preventing and managing depression and anxiety.

We've also gone over the top food categories to aid you in this fight. These are the food groups that have the highest nutrient density of the specific vitamins and minerals we know can both prevent and better manage the symptoms associated with mental health disorders. That said, how you integrate these different categories into your diet is entirely up to you. Pick the foods that appeal most to you and eat them in the way that aligns with your tastes and values. Considering these different categories, and the foods you enjoy the most within each of them, is the first step in tapping into a powerful new way to care for both your body and your brain.

But, as everyone knows, knowing and doing are two different things. That's why the following section of this book will help to guide you as you continue on this journey. We'll discuss the different challenges you may face as you make brain-boosting changes to your diet, as well as offer you different tools and tips to make it easier as you do so.

It isn't always straightforward or comfortable to delve more deeply into what may be driving your current food choices. Mental health conditions often change the way we think about ourselves, how we interact with our environments, and, by extension, the way we eat. Making changes to any routine, including your dietary pattern, can be a challenge. But the science is clear: food plays a vital role in promoting brain health and resilience. And it's one of the easiest components of treatment that can be entirely within your own control.

Moving forward, we'll discuss the best ways to prepare for the Eat to Beat Depression and Anxiety Six-Week Plan, a simple guide to increasing your intake of brain-healthy food categories. We will take a good look at your food roots, preferences, and many of the challenges that face modern eaters. We'll then delve into the plan itself, with best practices, strategies for common challenges, and recipes that highlight the principles and foods we've been discussing. My ultimate goal is for you to find ways to confidently and joyfully use food to empower you in your fight against depression and anxiety.

CHAPTER 5: Recap

- Eating to beat depression goes beyond eating a single "superfood" or simply trying to add a few extra nutrients into your diet. Rather, eating for brain health involves consuming whole foods with a high nutrient density provided directly by Mother Nature.

- To help you eat the foods you most enjoy, this book focuses on food categories, or groupings of different foods, that contain high levels of brain-healthy nutrients.

- Focusing on broader food categories helps make it easier to make simple swaps and substitutions to increase your nutrient density. Eating shouldn't be a chore—so pick the foods in each category that appeal most to you.

- The *Eat to Beat Depression and Anxiety* food categories are leafy greens; rainbow fruits and vegetables; seafood; nuts, beans, and seeds; meat; eggs and dairy; and good microbiome bugs.

- As anyone who has tried to change their diet can tell you, knowing and doing are two different things. You may know what foods are best for your health. But by using food categories, instead of a more prescriptive diet plan, you have the power to choose the foods you like to care for both your body and brain.

PART II

Get Started: Your Path to Healing

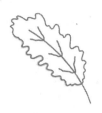

Chapter 6

· · · · · · ·

CHALLENGES FACING
THE MODERN EATER

Food is complicated for many, many different reasons.

We've already talked about how much food has changed in the United States over the past one hundred years, moving from local, farm-fresh foods to prepackaged convenience items. But, beyond those changes, an overwhelming form of diet culture also permeates almost every aspect of today's society. Consumers are constantly bombarded with confusing, conflicting, or just plain inaccurate information about foods and their influence on health and well-being. It's challenging enough just to sift through all that information—let alone figure out how you can effectively harness it to make positive changes to your diet.

Every year, there's a new trendy diet that hits the mainstream. You may notice this year's hot take on food will reverse the mainstays of last year's recommended guidelines. And, more often than not, the only thing that these different fad diets have in common is the message that you're somehow eating all wrong. The end result, for many people, is fear and shame. Fear that we don't understand how to eat properly to maintain optimal health, and shame that many of the things we enjoy may be highlighted on some sort of "bad" foods list.

Take Susan, for instance. When she came to see me, she had

some very strong ideas about what constituted healthy eating—but, even with such firmly held notions, she admitted she wasn't sure about how to properly nourish her brain.

"I read almost every article on diet and health I can find," she said. "This week, I read that I'm supposed to go keto and start eating a ketogenic diet. But then I read it's bad for my heart. Another article says eating vegan is the healthiest way to go. Then another will tell you that you need to eat goji berries or fast or do something else to be healthy. It's enough to make your head spin."

She's right—it is. And, for many people who struggle with anxiety, all the conflicting information makes them even more fretful about their food choices. They feel like this is something they just will never get *right*.

As we move forward, I want to reiterate that there is no one *right* way to eat to beat depression and anxiety. Your mileage may vary—and, given that your journey is like no one else's, that's the way it should be.

I'd like to say that diet culture is the only barrier to eating to beat depression and anxiety—but it's not. We all have different tastes, preferences, and societal factors that influence the way we like to—and actually do—nourish ourselves. Some of us are picky eaters by nature. Others may have been raised with religious or cultural guidelines that dictate we avoid certain foods. There are a variety of political and environmental values that may encourage us to embrace one diet over another one. And many of us are likely constrained by time, cost, or just plain, simple motivation to move away from convenience eating.

Susan's practice of regularly eating iceberg lettuce salads with chicken and cucumber was built on many of those personal values. It's a dish her mother taught her would help her stay "thin"—which, in her mind, was strongly associated with being healthy. As we talked about ways to easily add more nutrient-dense foods to her diet, it was important to address those kinds of beliefs, as well as other challenges she faced, to help empower her to make changes.

Without doing so, it would have been much harder for her to break such longstanding habits.

No matter which way you approach it, food is complicated—and a lot of people out there are trying to sell you on a particular diet. (Sometimes, literally—with specialized supplements promising miracles.) That's why it's so important to accept that some of the things we've been told about eating "healthy" can get in our way as we try to best nourish our brains. As I said earlier, this isn't a diet book, nor one that suggests simply changing up your diet as some kind of cure-all that will alleviate your need for other interventions like talk therapy or antidepressant medications. As a therapist, my goal is always to help my patients embrace progress, not perfection. To make that progress, it's important that you respect your unique tastes and values about food, which are as individual as your experiences with depression and anxiety.

When it comes to nutrition and the brain, there is no single "right" way to eat. In discussing the nutrients highlighted in the AFS, as well as the recommended food categories from the previous chapter, my aim is to help you understand the basic foundational building blocks that can truly nourish your brain. It's up to you to figure out what works best for you—and, because of that, you're much more likely to see positive, sustained changes to your mood and anxiety levels.

COMMON QUESTIONS ABOUT EATING TO BEAT DEPRESSION AND ANXIETY

I understand that it can be difficult to change ingrained habits regarding what and how you eat, especially when you aren't feeling your best. I also understand that we all face a variety of hurdles that sometimes make eating to beat depression and anxiety more challenging than it needs to be. That's why in this chapter, I'll address some of the most common questions I receive from patients, as well as the audiences I speak to, about different dietary challenges to better prepare you to fully participate in Chapter 9's six-week plan.

Chances are, one of the questions discussed below is an obstacle to you finding your own way to becoming a master of self-nourishment. By tackling such challenges head on, it's my hope that you can better build both confidence and joy to make the sorts of small dietary changes and substitutions that can work to big effect in improving your mood and anxiety levels.

Can't I just take supplements?

For the last hundred years, many Americans have relied on a daily multivitamin to increase levels of certain vitamins and minerals. Supplements can be helpful in restoring nutrient deficiencies, of course—your physician may have even prescribed some to you—but multivitamins and other supplements cannot fully replace the nutritional value of good old-fashioned food. A number of studies have shown that multivitamins simply don't provide enough of the necessary nutrients to be effective—and, as such, a daily vitamin wasn't linked to positive improvements in health. That's one of the reasons why the U.S. Preventive Services Task Force (USPSTF)—an independent panel of health experts that reviews the effectiveness of preventative medications, tests, and procedures—doesn't recommend supplements to help prevent or manage disease.

There are several reasons why supplements can't compete with food. The first is a matter of absorption. The body was designed to absorb vital nutrients from food. Common minerals like calcium, magnesium, and iron can actually block others from being taken up into the body through the gut. When two or more are packed into pill form, it's more than likely that you won't absorb as much of them.

Second, many of the phytonutrients that are found in rainbow fruits, vegetables, and leafy greens are difficult to put into supplement form. The sulforaphane you get from fresh spinach is going to be very different from what you get from the dehydrated food concentrates commonly found packed in vitamin pills.

Finally, many supplements are contaminated with other ingredients that can lead to adverse reactions. Supplements do not need FDA approval and are not monitored or tested with the same scrutiny as medications. Over the years, different vitamin brands have been recalled for containing heavy metals, like lead or cadmium, or adulterants that may trigger allergies. While popping a multivitamin each morning may be easy, it won't give you the complete nourishment your brain needs to stay healthy and strong.

However, there are some supplements I do sometimes recommend. For example, some people need to take a vitamin D supplement as low levels are quite common and you should get yours checked by your physician annually. Over the years I've prescribed magnesium, St. John's wort, melatonin, L-methylfolate, and many others. But I often meet patients who are taking a number of supplements without much clear effect—and remember, our body must deal with whatever we consume. Processing megadoses of vitamins, minerals, herbs, and often additives (and even toxins like cadmium, lead, and pharmaceutical analogs) is hard work for the liver and kidneys.

I should also add that there are synergistic relationships between the nutrients you find in different foods. As I've said before, many of these nutrients travel together—and for good reason. Mother Nature knew what she was doing. That's why olive oil is such powerful food for brain health. It helps your body absorb those vital fat-soluble nutrients like vitamin A and the phytonutrient lycopene. Supplements just can't compete with that.

That said, the main reason I favor food over supplements has to do with pleasure. You can't experiment and come up with new recipes with vitamin pills. There's no sitting down and savoring a meal of protein shakes with friends and family. No one has ever taken a supplement and thought, "Wow, that tasted amazing!" A life fueled solely by powders, shakes, and pills just isn't all that nourishing, for your body or your spirit.

As anyone who has sat down to a meal full of good food and laughter knows, what we eat is meant to be enjoyed. When we reduce food to just a set of nutrients, further distancing ourselves from our social networks and the greater food system, we lose more than just taste. We lose a way to connect to friends, family, and the world around us. We lose our ability to connect with ourselves. To my mind, as we think about the nutrients that can truly nourish our brains, that knowledge should inspire us to head to the places where we can get fresh, whole foods that sate both our bodies and our souls—not just take a trip to the pharmacy's vitamin aisle.

Is junk food really *that* bad?

Having the occasional treat is never a bad thing. I happen to have a sweet tooth myself. The problem comes when the majority of your diet comes from processed foods. You have to eat no matter what. So, when you aren't consuming nutrient-dense foods, you're instead filling up on foods that are likely to have a negative impact on your health. The occasional bag of chips or chocolate chip cookie won't get in the way of eating to beat depression. But when you rely too heavily on convenience foods or junk foods for your meals, you leave a gap in nutrients that is nearly impossible to fill.

Will eating from these food categories help me lose weight? Or gain weight?

Too often depression, anxiety, and weight issues go hand in hand. Some people experience significant weight gain while others may lose weight to an unhealthy degree. Medications used to treat these conditions can cause weight gain, as can the food habits that come with emotional eating. So, as you can imagine, many of my patients ask me about how changing their dietary pattern might affect the number they see on the scale.

Weight fluctuations in depression happen for a variety of different reasons and depend greatly on an individual's current diet and how much they exercise. Chapter 9's six-week plan is not meant to be a weight loss regimen; it's a protocol meant to help you build a stronger, more resilient brain. That said, many people who follow the plan do end up seeing some weight loss as they swap out processed foods for more whole foods like fresh seafood and vegetables.

What if I have food allergies or food sensitivities?

Many of the brain-boosting power players, including shellfish, eggs, and nuts, also happen to top the list of common food allergens. When exposed to them, some people may experience a mild rash or some tummy troubles—but others may respond to these allergens with significant bowel issues or even anaphylactic shock.

Food allergies are another reason why I wanted to move away from specific recommended foods to broader categories. For example, a person may be allergic to cashews but not pumpkin seeds. However, if you have a food allergy, proceed with caution. Often you can pick another food in that category with a similar nutrient profile to replace it. But, before doing so, I recommend speaking with your healthcare providers for their recommendations about your safest options.

In other cases, you may not be allergic to a particular food but have an increased sensitivity to it. Perhaps, after consuming it, you experience bloating or gas, or maybe you feel extra amped up or even really tired. Whatever it is, when you eat that food, you just don't feel good. The good news is, you don't have to eat it. That's another reason why I advocate for food categories. If there's a food that doesn't agree with you for whatever reason, there are plenty of other options that also contain the nutrients you need. As you go through the categories, take careful note of what works for you—and then select the foods that make you feel the best.

What if I don't like green vegetables?

You're not alone! In fact, nearly 15 percent of people are what are called "supertasters." Their taste buds are particularly attuned to the bitterness of greens—and, as such, they just don't enjoy eating them. There's quite a lot that can be done to counter that bitter taste, and many of my patients have found successful ways to add greens to their diets.

Try to use baby greens instead of the adult varieties. You can get your greens in the late fall, after the season's first frost, as it tends to sweeten them. Try different types—you might find watercress, red cabbage, or red lettuce to be more tolerable than kale or arugula. If those greens are still a bit too unpleasant for you, the addition of a few key spices, or sautéing your greens with onions or garlic, can really change the flavor. You can also throw greens and other veggies into soups or stews to help temper the taste. There's a leafy green out there for you. It just may take a bit of experimenting to find the one that works with your taste buds.

Others may experience issues with the texture of not only greens but also other vegetables. They just don't like the way these foods feel in their mouths. Again, here's a place where adding extra veggies to soups and stews, as well as adding them to smoothies or other blends, can help make all sorts of great nutrient-dense veggies more palatable even to the pickiest of eaters.

Should I have concerns about eating seafood?

Consuming more seafood—or any seafood at all, for that matter—can be a challenge for a variety of reasons. It certainly was for me. As a farm boy from Indiana, the only fish I regularly ate growing up were the fish sticks in the school cafeteria. With my main seafood experience the smell of those sticks, was it any wonder I spent most of my life thinking I despised seafood?

Once the evidence started piling up about the link between omega-3s and brain health—as well as studies demonstrating that people who regularly ate seafood were less likely to have issues with either depression or anxiety—I knew I had to get past my aversion. I had to learn how to eat seafood because it's one of the only sources of those amazing long-chain omega-3 fats. I managed to do so by trying different varieties of fish, prepared in a range of different ways. It took some time, but I got there.

While you may not be haunted by the memory of soggy fish sticks, it's possible that you just don't like the taste of seafood. For some, its "fishy" taste can be difficult to get past. Because seafood contains high levels of polyunsaturated fatty acids, it can spoil much more quickly than beef or chicken. Buying fresh-caught seafood, when available, is always your best bet. Good seafood should both smell and taste of the sea, but not "fishy"—and milder white fish easily takes on the flavor of your favorite sauces and seasonings.

Even if you adore the taste of salmon or oysters, so-called fishier fishes like mackerel may still be difficult. (Hint: Add ginger.) It's a misnomer that popular shellfish like mussels and clams are "bottom" feeders. They are filter feeders, collecting their nutrients by filtering them out of the seawater as it moves through their shells. That style of feeding, however, doesn't make them dirty or unhealthy to eat.

Then there are religious considerations. For example, those who keep kosher aren't supposed to eat any seafood that lacks fins and scales. That knocks shrimp, oysters, and lobster—just to name a few—off the list.

Finally, many patients have come to me with concerns about contaminants in seafood, either heavy metals, mercury, or microplastics. Nearly twenty years ago, scientists started to see that both ocean and freshwater fish had alarmingly high levels of mercury and persistant organic pollutants, like flame retardants and plastics. Fish and shellfish, because of the way their physiology is set up, tend to take in and concentrate heavy metals from polluted waters. Since high levels of mercury can be dangerous, this is, certainly, of great concern. Similarly, increased water pollution also means that many fish are now ingesting tiny pieces of plastic, or microplastics, that stay in their bodies over time—and, as such, eventually end up on our plates. Generally you can avoid both mercury and microplastics by serving up smaller fish like anchovies or sardines, or instead enjoying bivalve shellfish like clams and mussels.

Seafood is a fairly broad food category. If you're looking for ideas on how to best expand your palate, be a little adventurous and try the seafood special at your favorite restaurant—or ask your local fishmonger for recommendations for what's most fresh and flavorful.

Isn't eating red meat bad for your heart?

Over the past two years, there have been a lot of studies looking at the effects of red meat on health—including beef, lamb, and processed meat. The consistent message has been that red meat is linked to heart disease and inflammation; there have even been some studies that suggest consuming high amounts of red meat may even be linked to cancer.[1] Historically, these links have been attributed to the saturated fats and cholesterol found in meat—as well as the high amounts of beef that the average American eats each week.

On top of those studies, many are also concerned about the environmental impact of eating meat. Large-scale beef production isn't the most humane of enterprises, and the way many operations turn out beef products raises serious sustainability issues. These methods of beef production can also lead to a higher saturated fat profile in the meat. Is it any wonder that so many people are considering vegetarian or even vegan diets? Or, at the very least, just want to limit their beef intake?

As a former vegetarian, I'm here to tell you that it's possible to eat meat healthfully, ethically, and responsibly—and that it can be a great advantage to do so as you're eating to beat depression and anxiety. Several studies have found links between vegetarian diets and depressive symptoms, especially in men. And a study published in the *European Journal of Clinical Nutrition* found that vegans tend to be significantly deficient in vitamin B12. As B12 is one of the key nutrients on the AFS—and isn't found in plants— that's of concern.

That said, you don't have to trade heart health for brain health. You don't have to give up your ethical principles regarding the environment, either. There's a happy medium to be had when you consider how to best integrate red meat into your diet. First, when choosing your cuts of meat, opt for grass-fed products. They tend to have a very different fat profile than their grain-fed counterparts; lower in overall fat and containing more monounsaturated, omega-3, and CLA fats linked to health. Buy from smaller, family-owned farms that put quality first. This, too, better guarantees the quality of the meat you and your family will consume and also puts less of a strain on the environment.

In addition, it's important to stop thinking about meat as the main part of your meal. Felice Jacka, the researcher who led the SMILES trial, found that the amount of red meat you eat matters— and matters quite a bit when you consider both heart and brain health. Back in 2012, she and her colleagues looked at red meat intake and depression in one thousand adult women. They discovered an interesting trend. Women who regularly ate more than the recommended daily intake were more likely to be depressed. Perhaps that wasn't so much of a surprise. Yet, she and her colleagues also discovered that women who consistently consumed *less* than the recommended amounts were also more likely to be depressed—and that's after controlling for every other factor that she and her team could think of. After grokking the numbers from the study, Jacka found that eating a moderate amount of lean red meat—no more than two pounds per week—can be a boon to brain health. As such, when you eat meat sparingly, as a way to flavor the veggies and grains that should make up the bulk of your meal, you can be confident you are doing so with both heart and brain health in mind.

But I'm not interested in giving up my vegan/vegetarian lifestyle.

No problem! As I said earlier, eating for brain health can be done in a variety of different ways. I know that a lot of people are committed to living a vegetarian or vegan lifestyle. You still have the power to eat to beat depression and anxiety; you just need to look carefully at different options within each of the food categories to make sure you're getting critical brain health nutrients like polyunsaturated fatty acids and vitamin B12. I'll be honest: it's harder when you don't eat seafood or meat but certainly not impossible.

One way to increase your B12 is through purple nori, a type of seaweed—and, coincidentally, the reason why I consider seaweed to be a power-player food. This purple sea plant, often sold in a dried form at your favorite Asian food store, contains several different types of biologically active B12 compounds. When researchers from Japan's Hagoromo-Gakuen College gave B12-deficient rats this superfood, they were able to significantly improve their status.[2] And those positive effects aren't limited to rodents. A review from researchers from Tottori University, also in Japan, highlighted purple nori as a great source of vital nutrients, from vitamin B12 to iron, for those who don't want to include meat in their diet.[3]

Can I get the nutrients I need from chicken?

Many people use chicken as their go-to protein. I get it: it's versatile, tasty, and lighter than beef. That said, while a serving of lean chicken breast does have about half the recommended daily allowance for vitamin B6 and selenium, it doesn't have the same kind of nutrient punch as red meat.

What about eggs?

Depending on what year you were born, you may remember the old advertising slogan about the "incredible, edible egg." Others may have been raised with the notion that eggs are high in cholesterol and should be limited, if not outright avoided, if you're trying to maintain a healthy diet. The truth of the matter is that eggs really are a perfect brain food, filled to the brim with B vitamins, including AFS notables like B6, B12, and folate. They're chock-full of vitamin D and contain magnesium, zinc, and iron, too. Eggs are an excellent protein source and house those important omega-3 fatty acids our brains rely on. They really are a nutrient powerhouse and can be a key player in your strategy to beat depression or anxiety.

Eggs also contain choline, a close cousin of the B-vitamin family, which has been linked to the prevention and management of anxiety symptoms. It works by helping to support learning and memory processes by providing the building blocks for myelin, that important brain insulation, as well as several key neurotransmitters.

As for dietary cholesterol, eggs aren't as big of a health villain as we were led to believe. One, although they do contain a high amount of cholesterol, the body doesn't absorb most of it. So, unless you're frying up a few dozen eggs a day to include in your meals, having one for breakfast or as an afternoon pick-me-up shouldn't negatively affect your lipid panel.

Like red meat, some people have ethical concerns about eating eggs. But, again, I believe it's possible to eat them in a healthy and sustainable manner. With so many egg options on grocery shelves—grade A, pasture-raised, free-range, organic, cage-free— it can be hard to know which are healthiest. For the most part, there's not much difference in nutritional quality. When you can, buy eggs from a local farmer who lets the birds roam free. Those are likely to be the most nutrient dense, with higher levels of omega-3s. But if that option is not available to you, grabbing a carton of organic, pasture-raised, or cage-free eggs at the store will make sure you have access to a remarkable source of brain-boosting nutrients.

You know, I've heard a lot of the same things about dairy.

Milk, cheese, and butter are other foods that are often heavily debated in nutritional circles. And, over the years, the resounding message has been that these foods are full of "bad" saturated fats that can lead to heart disease.

You've heard me say, on more than one occasion, that fat is not the enemy. I'm going to repeat it here. Because fat really isn't your enemy. It, too, plays a vital role in promoting brain health. Dairy is full of nutrients, including different fats that help to keep your brain cells in tip-top shape—especially products made from grass-fed ruminants.

Many people gravitate toward processed "cheese products"— those old prepackaged holdovers from childhood. These products are full of hydrogenated oils as well as artificial colorings and flavorings. Frankly, these products are often more other stuff than actual cheese. With a category as diverse as dairy, there are so many different options to try beyond the cow. For example, why not try a really amazing goat or sheep cheese? I heartily recommended visiting your local farmers market and talking to the cheesemonger about different options that appeal to your taste buds.

One of the main things dairy has going for it is its different fermented options. Yogurt and kefir both provide great food for the microbiome, which we know promotes brain health. For individuals who are lactose intolerant, fermented dairy eliminates most of this form of dairy sugar, making it easier to digest and enjoy. But I'd caution you to read the labels on the different products you find in the refrigerated aisle before taking them home. Many popular yogurt brands are nothing more than glorified sugar bombs—and even flavored kefirs can be chock-full of added sweeteners. Your best bet is to find plain, whole-milk varieties of both and then add in your own sweetness with a handful of berries, some honey, or a little dark chocolate.

Speaking of sugar . . .

There's been a lot of talk in the media about the dangers of sugar consumption—and for good reason. The average American consumes an alarming amount of sugar. According to the American Heart Association, the recommended maximum of added sugar should be between 6 and 9 teaspoons *a day*. The average American consumes 22 teaspoons of added sugar per day.[4] Yes, you read that right. Most of us eat far more than that without even realizing it—in fact, some people manage that in just a couple cups of coffee.

It's amazing how much sugar is in a can of soda pop or a fancy coffee.

New studies, like the Whitehall II study, have demonstrated that those who consume high amounts of sugar are more likely to be diagnosed with a mood or other mental health disorder.[5] That's why it's important to take a hard look at some of the foods you eat. Many convenience items are chock-full of sugar, and even many products that are marketed as "healthy" or "organic," contain more than their fair share of refined sugar. As you start to think about the best ways to eat to beat depression and anxiety, it's critical to remember that too much sugar can work against you.

There are certainly plenty of sugar substitutes out there—and many people rely on artificial sweeteners like Equal or NutraSweet to augment the taste of everything from coffee to baked goods. I'd just add a word of caution: the use of such sweeteners over time has the power to alter your palate. Simply put, they may trick your taste buds into thinking you are getting a little sugar, but they don't fool your brain. Repeated use of artificial sweeteners, like downing a few diet sodas every day, can lead to people consuming more sugary foods, and therefore a lot more empty calories, than they otherwise would.

Sugar and carbohydrate cravings are among the most common concerns I've heard from eaters. It's important to remember that not all carbohydrates are created equal. Focus on "slow-burning" carbs in plants and whole grains. Here are some healthy swaps next time you get hit with a snack attack.

Should I be fasting? What about trying the keto diet?

Anecdotal evidence suggests both of these new diets may be of some benefit to mental health—and there are a few studies that support the idea. Many animal studies have now looked at intermittent fasting, or restricting food for sixteen hours each day, and discovered it can help protect the brain from a variety of stressors

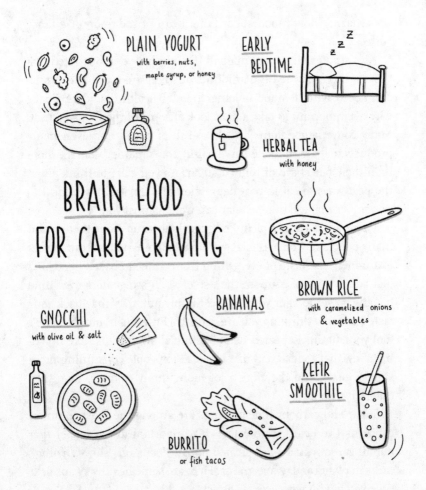

PLAIN YOGURT
with berries, nuts,
maple syrup, or honey

EARLY
BEDTIME

HERBAL TEA
with honey

BRAIN FOOD
FOR CARB CRAVING

BROWN RICE
with caramelized onions
& vegetables

BANANAS

GNOCCHI
with olive oil & salt

KEFIR
SMOOTHIE

BURRITO
or fish tacos

ranging from oxidative stress to stroke. Similarly, ketogenic diets, with their high-protein/high-fat regimen, encourage the body to burn fats instead of carbohydrates, which can also help optimize brain function. While both are gaining popularity across the country—and I've had a few patients who've found success with them—the human studies have been quite limited in both scope and time. The data really isn't there yet.

I'd also add that these are really challenging diets to maintain.

Trying to figure out the right balance of protein to carbohydrates to get into a state of ketosis is a lot of work. And for many, especially those who may be struggling with depressive or anxiety symptoms, trying to manage intermittent fasting is equally burdensome. If you're interested in fasting or keto, please talk to your healthcare provider to help you determine a safe, healthy way forward.

You aren't going to try to take my coffee away, are you?

I know many of us rely on that initial jolt of caffeine each morning to get up and get moving. Just as I'd like you to start eating a larger variety of rainbow vegetables, I'd also like you to consider where else you might get your morning pick-me-up. There are so many amazing green and black teas out there—and, chances are, there's one that you will enjoy as much as your coffee. So why not mix it up a little? Teas also come with a number of health benefits, since they're chock-full of antioxidants and polyphenols. And while many varieties also contain caffeine, they tend to contain less than your average cup of joe.

For those of you struggling with anxiety, I think it's important to take a long, hard look at your caffeine intake. There's a reason why you rely on that shot of caffeine to wake up—it's a stimulant. As such, too much caffeine has been known to promote anxious feelings and even, in some cases, anxiety attacks. Replacing coffee with an herbal tea or other noncaffeinated beverage may better serve you as you eat to beat anxiety.

Should I be eliminating grains or gluten from my diet?

I get this question a lot. Approximately 1 percent of the population has celiac disease, an inherited autoimmune disorder that makes the immune system attack the small intestine as it tries to digest gluten, which is a protein found in wheat, rye, and barley. This was a disease that, for a long time, was largely unknown and is still highly underdiagnosed—and, as such, it's gotten a lot of attention in recent years. Although, that said, it is a fairly rare condition.

Some individuals may also be sensitive or intolerant to gluten. About 200,000 people each year will be diagnosed with gluten sensitivity. They don't have as severe of an immune reaction to the protein, but eating it will result in some inflammation in the lower gut that can lead to diarrhea, bloating, gas, or fatigue. People with gluten and other food sensitivities often experience rashes, head-aches, joint aches, and mood changes. These symptoms are quite variable, and range from pretty uncomfortable to over time leading to some serious health consequences.

Eliminating gluten or other grains may be helpful to you, but for most people gluten or grains aren't the root cause of depres-sion and anxiety. Some people benefit from eliminating grains not from the gluten per se, but from eliminating the empty calories of pasta, bread, crackers, and pastries. You know your body best—and maybe wheat just doesn't work for you. That's okay, because there are lots of amazing grains out there to choose from, many of which are completely gluten free. Rice, quinoa, amaranth, oats, and buckwheat are all great options. They also have the added bonus of being incredibly nutrient dense. I'd recommend adding them to your pantry even if you aren't gluten intolerant.

Of course, some of us are just suckers for a great slice of bread. Today, it's easy to find artisanal breads made from whole grains, nuts, and seeds that can help you embrace foods from different cat-egories. There's even sourdough bread, its unique taste thanks to a fermentation process in the dough that helps to feed all those good bugs in your microbiome. Once you start thinking beyond sliced white bread, you'll find there's a whole world of grains that easily complement your favorite brain-boosting foods.

Isn't eating this way super expensive?

It's easy to think so, especially since most items marketed as healthy on supermarket shelves tend to come with a dollar or two markup in price. Yet, eating for brain health does not need to break the bank. Remember the SMILES trial? Many of the recommended food categories, like leafy greens and rainbow vegetables, are actually a great bargain. You can buy a big bunch of greens for only a few dollars. They last in the fridge all week—and you can even freeze them. Many prepackaged convenience foods end up being much, much pricier. That may be why, when Felice Jacka and her colleagues looked at the costs of moving to a brain-healthy diet during the SMILES trial, they found the study participants, on average, saved about $25 each week on their food purchases.

"So many brain-healthy foods are actually quite inexpensive," said Jacka. "When we did a cost analysis, and looked in great detail at what people were spending on food each month, the averages of what they were spending when they came into the study were actually higher than the costs of the diet we were advocating. Our diet was not only healthier but cheaper."

I fully understand why costs are a concern, especially as fresh produce can spoil much more quickly than processed or canned vegetables. But many foods, like whole grains, cheeses, nuts, and legumes are cheaper when purchased whole—and in bulk. A membership at a retail warehouse club can help your dollar stretch further when buying your favorite pantry staples.

A little bit of preparation can also help you save money. By planning out your meals in advance and using batch cooking techniques to use up fresh items before they go bad, you can make whole, fresh fruits and veggies go the distance.

You may also find some savings by shopping outside traditional grocery stores. Community supported agricultural (CSA) programs can provide you with a large carton of fresh, seasonal fruits and veggies each week for a reasonable price—and some insurance programs even provide rebates for your participation. If you already take part in a share, you know how large these weekly boxes can be. Many people will go in with a friend or family member to make the investment even more budget friendly. There are also opportunities to sign up for services that will regularly send you "imperfect" produce. For 20 to 30 percent less than grocery store prices, you can get fresh fruits and veggies that may not win any beauty contests but are just as fresh, wholesome, and delicious as their prettier counterparts.

It may take a little extra effort, but eating to beat depression and anxiety can be done on a budget. Once you start making substitutions and switches, I think you'll find your weekly grocery bill will remain on par with what it currently is.

GETTING YOURSELF READY

I'll say it again: food is complicated. Know that you're not alone in facing the challenges of adapting your diet to better serve your mental health.

As we move on to the next chapter, I'd like you to think about which obstacles you may be facing when it comes to different foods. Look more deeply into your current eating choices and why you tend to go for the foods you do. Both depression and anxiety have the power to change the way we think about ourselves and our environment—and, as such, the way we feed ourselves. But you don't need to approach food with fear or shame. Doing so only makes it harder to make changes to your diet.

As you start to think about the best ways to incorporate the different food categories to help you eat to beat depression and anxiety, it's essential to carefully assess where you are—and, more important, where you want to go. Moving forward, we'll take time to look at your relationship with food, as well as what motivates your food choices. By working from that place of understanding, you can better learn how to make sustainable, healthy changes that will support optimal brain health in the future. Let's dive in.

CHAPTER 6: Recap

- Food is complicated. Each and every day, consumers are bombarded with confusing, conflicting, and just plain inaccurate information about what they should be eating. But when it comes to making food choices for mental health, there's no one "right" way.
- As you approach Chapter 9's six-week plan, it's important to ask yourself questions and consider some of the challenges you may face as you start to incorporate more brain-healthy foods into your diet.
- Common questions and challenges regarding eating for brain nourishment include concerns about supplementation, food allergies, contaminants in seafood, meat and heart health, sugar, fasting, caffeine, and the costs involved with this way of eating.

Chapter 7

EATER, HEAL THYSELF

Nourishment Beyond Nutrients: Key
Lessons from the Brain Food Clinic

The way I treat depression in my clinical practice has radically changed over the last ten years. It all started with the converging evidence that food truly is medicine—and can help promote brain health and therefore better prevent and manage mental health conditions. Further, the way I used this information continued to evolve, as I listened to my patients who faced challenges as they tried to alter their diets. There were quite a few of them—and they needed to be acknowledged before more forward progress could be made.

My goal as a clinician is to help you build a more joyful and nourishing relationship with food. I can't just tell you to "eat better" or to simply add some kale to your breakfast sandwich. It's not that simple. You can't just tell people to do something. Rather, it's critical to take the time to carefully consider what may be getting in the way of reaching your goal of empowering yourself to choose healthy, nutrient-dense foods—and, in the process, gain the knowledge, skills, and confidence you need to eat to beat depression and anxiety. That's why I founded the Brain Food Clinic in New York City. I wanted to be able to incorporate evidence-based nutrition and integrative psychiatry treatments with more traditional therapies to help people lead more joyful, fulfilled lives.

In the last chapter, you read some of the common questions I hear both from my patients and the audiences I speak to about the importance of choosing the right foods to nourish your brain. Like I said, food is complicated. And, unfortunately, thanks to a variety of factors, many of us end up making it even more complicated than it needs to be. Maybe you relate to some of the challenges addressed in the previous pages, or maybe you're facing different hurdles to changing your dietary pattern. Either way, taking the time to carefully assess your personal relationship with food is the next step to better understand the links between food and your mental health, as well as to identify how, where, and when to set specific, achievable, and sustainable goals to address them. The power to make change lies solely within you.

In my practice, patients work closely with me or my colleague Samantha Elkrief, LMSW—a therapist, health coach, and chef—to do a food assessment. Then, based on what we discover together, we come up with an appropriate action plan. These assessments are a crucial part of how we develop our treatment plans. They are all about diving into the nitty-gritty of what a person eats, discovering the foods they most enjoy, what they are already doing well, and identifying opportunities to make small, positive changes.

"So often, people have the information they need to eat for brain health, but they get a little stuck when it comes time to try to actually make a change to their meals or snacks," says Elkrief. "For many people, what might be blocking them isn't immediately obvious. It takes asking the right questions for them to see, 'Oh, this is a pattern,' or 'I didn't realize this was an issue for me.' That's the value of doing this kind of assessment."

You don't need to set up an appointment with us to reap the benefits of a food assessment. Instead, you complete your own at home by answering some simple questions.

As you start to go through the questions, please remember that this exercise isn't about judgment or shame. The questionnaire isn't meant to make you feel bad, or even worse, to make you think you're attempting the impossible—quite the opposite, in fact. This type of assessment is about exploring your relationship with food so you can take small steps forward. Again, it's about progress, not perfection. While it's important to acknowledge your challenges around food and change, the focus should be on finding the tools and motivation you need to make smart changes and keep them going long-term.

Often, I find people already have a good idea about where they need to make improvements when it comes to diet. Trust your gut on that one. But, just as often, there may be challenges that aren't as immediately apparent. This is a place where you can sit down, consider what may be holding you back, and put a name to your obstacles. That way you can be sure they're addressed once you start Chapter 9's six-week plan.

While food is complicated, this assessment doesn't have to be. Just answer the questions honestly—and then walk through the details of what you eat each day. You will likely find, by writing down what you eat, you'll start thinking about it differently. Then, you can better identify the patterns within your regular eating habits that work for you—and those that may need to be reconsidered. From there, you can develop the skills and define the small, specific goals that will get you where you need to be. Remember: progress, not perfection. Eating to beat depression and anxiety happens one meal, one food, and one bite at a time.

WHY ARE YOU HERE?

There's a reason why you picked up this book. That's the first thing I'd like you to think about as you prepare to start the six-week plan.

In the psychiatry world, we would call this defining a patient's "chief complaint." Think about the following questions:

- Have you or a loved one been diagnosed with depression or anxiety?
- If so, what are the primary symptoms?
- What most concerns you about preventing or managing symptoms related to these disorders?
- What are your primary concerns regarding your mental health and when did they start?
- What is bothering you the most—and has gotten you to the point where you are ready to make some changes?
- If food were to help you beat depression and anxiety, what would that look like for you?

Remember Pete, the twentysomething man who came to me for treatment of his recurring depression? From the outside, many people might have thought that Pete was most bothered by the fact that he was once again living with his parents or out of work. From the outside, failure to launch looks like it would be a significant source of disappointment. But Pete's primary reason for seeking treatment was more about how he felt on the inside—"Down and pretty dark" most of the time. His number one goal was to regain energy levels, to find pleasure in the activities he used to enjoy so much, and just plain feel better.

"I just don't have much energy to do anything," he said. "It sometimes feels like nothing I used to like to do is really all that worthwhile anymore. I'd like that to change."

Whether you, like Pete, are hoping to increase your energy levels or just want to do a better job of nourishing your family, understanding the whys can help you determine your best next steps. They can also help identify potential challenges you may have as you seek to embrace more food categories in your meal planning.

WHAT IS YOUR RELATIONSHIP WITH FOOD?

Maybe you were a member of the clean plate club as a kid—and, today, you don't feel like you've finished a meal unless you feel incredibly full. Perhaps food is tightly intertwined with the culture in which you were raised. You associate feelings of comfort with a big bowl of pasta or a freshly baked cake. It's possible you were raised in a family that cooks everything from scratch. The thought of a boxed meal makes you turn up your nose. Alternatively, you may have grown up in a home where you, even from a young age, were expected to make your own meals while your parents worked. As such, your strongest kitchen skill remains the ability to push buttons on the microwave. Each and every one of us has a relationship with food—and it plays a fundamental role in how we nourish ourselves.

As you may recall, Susan was raised eating fairly basic iceberg lettuce salads. She was told they were healthy and would help her keep her weight under control. As she considered her own relationship with food, she realized how much of what she did revolved around some form of deprivation—and how that affected her feelings of anxiety and worry. She also struggled with the idea that there was a "right" way to feed herself and that she, for the most part, was doing things incorrectly. As we talked more about her relationship with food, there was something else I learned about Susan. Her mother didn't cook. As such, Susan hadn't spent much time cooking herself. She felt a keen lack of confidence when it came to even basic skills in the kitchen.

"We do a lot of takeout, to be honest. I can heat things up in the microwave, of course. And I can chop up veggies with the best of them," she said. "But that's about the extent of it."

Understanding this aspect of her relationship with food gave Susan a good idea of where to start making simple, stress-free substitutions. It doesn't take much skill to toss some fruit, greens, and kefir into a blender for a nutrient-dense smoothie. Hard-boiling eggs was also well within her cooking repertoire. And with Susan's chopping skills, she was also in a great place to start making a folate-rich pesto that both she and her family would come to love to eat.

As you think about your relationship with food, ask yourself the following questions (note: we've found that our patients can better address these questions when they take time to journal about the answers):

- What was food like when you were growing up?
- Did your family eat together? What did that mean to you?
- What kinds of foods did your family prepare? Did you prepare them together?
- Where do you get your food today? From work? From school? Does your spouse or someone else prepare it for you?
- Do you feel comfortable cooking?
- What about eating at restaurants?
- What percentage of your meals are home-cooked? How often do you eat out?
- What are your go-to foods? What foods satisfy you the most? What foods bring you the most comfort?
- How do you feel shopping for healthy foods at the grocery store?
- How are your skills in the kitchen?
- What's one aspect of your relationship to food and one kitchen skill that you'd like to improve?

By taking this inventory, you can better understand your history, habits, and how to impact your personal relationship with food. Doing so can help highlight challenges regarding your food choices that you might not have considered before—but, more important, this can help you identify opportunities for change.

Often, our histories show us where we're comfortable. For example, if you grew up eating a lot of different types of food, you may be more open-minded about trying new things. If you grew up eating things in a single way, you may not realize that food can be cooked in a better way. The frozen microwavable veggies your mom served might not have been to your taste, but then you try some amazing roasted brussels sprouts and realize you actually do enjoy green vegetables. By understanding where you come from, you can identify and then create opportunities for change—and feel more confident about making small moves to help those changes happen.

WHAT'S YOUR DIETARY PATTERN?

Understanding your current dietary pattern is all about knowing what you eat on a regular basis. Ask yourself the following:

- What's your typical breakfast?
- What's your typical lunch?
- What's your typical dinner?
- Do you snack? If so, what do you typically eat?
- Do you eat small meals throughout the day? Or just three larger meals?
- What are your favorite foods?
- What are your problem foods?
- What are your go-to beverages? What do you drink each day?
- Do you have any food allergies or sensitivities?
- What about strong aversions?
- What are your strongest food categories? Where are you already succeeding?

While you may think you can easily answer these questions off the top of your head, experience tells us that people often miss important patterns or hurdles when they try to rely solely on memory. Instead, we heartily recommend journaling everything you eat for at least an entire week. You can grab a notebook to jot down your intake and observations. Think about it during your commute as you travel between home and work. Or, alternatively, there are now a number of great food journal apps that you can download to your smartphone or other favorite electronic device. In our clinic, we recommend finding whatever medium makes it easiest for you to consistently and accurately keep track of what you're eating. It's important not to overthink it.

After each meal or snack, write down exactly what you ate and when you ate it. Be honest: remember, this exercise is for you to understand when and what you're eating. This will offer insights into where you can make changes. It's not about judgment or to make you feel bad about your choices. It's there to show you where you are. As we often see in clinical practice, this initial food journal really helps open people's eyes about their eating habits. This information along with a few notes about how well you slept, as well as a 1 to 10 rating for your mood and anxiety levels for the day,

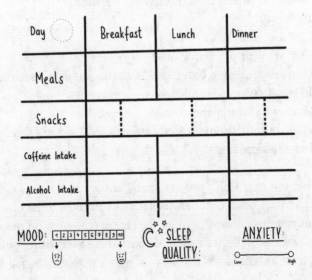

can also be of help. We've included a simple food journal to help get you started.

By taking the time to document what you're eating over the period of a week, the patterns become more apparent. You may notice you tend to feel a bit of an energy crash midafternoon and immediately grab some chips or a sugary snack from a vending machine. This is a great spot for a substitution. If you recognize you have this midday slump, you can make sure you have some nuts or maybe a piece of fruit on hand to eat instead. Alternatively, you may see that you're always grabbing a donut on your way into work when you're running late. Having hard-boiled eggs on hand in your fridge will allow you to grab a high-protein bite for breakfast even when you're in a rush.

You may see that, by the end of the week, you're gravitating toward lasagna. Maybe that's a comfort food for you—and that's not a bad thing! It's something you enjoy. But it also offers you one of those opportunities for change. You love lasagna. But could you add more veggies or greens to it? Can you add more of the nutrients your brain needs? Acknowledging that this is an important meal for you gives you something you can think about and work with.

Journaling isn't just about noticing places for improvement. It also offers you the ability to document and celebrate all the ways you're already succeeding in eating to beat depression and anxiety.

"Often, patients will come in after journaling for a week and say, 'Wow, I ate greens every day!' Or, 'I actually eat a lot of rainbow fruits and veggies.' Until they wrote it down, they honestly didn't realize they were doing so well in one category or another," says Elkrief. "When you are struggling with depression or anxiety, it can sometimes feel like you aren't doing anything all that well. But the journal can show you places where you are already achieving success. It gives you a tangible sense of where you really are when it comes to your diet."

CONSIDER YOUR MOTIVATIONS

Now that you've defined your primary concerns, relationship with food, and dietary pattern, it's time to take into account your motivations for wanting to make a change. What's really driving you to do so?

Psychologists talk a lot about intrinsic and extrinsic motivation. Intrinsic motivation is making changes because doing so is rewarding to you in some way, while extrinsic motivation is making a change for some outside reason—maybe to avoid a punishment or earn some type of reward.

So ask yourself, why are you motivated to eat to beat depression and anxiety? What's your end goal here?

Making changes to your dietary pattern isn't easy. We've certainly talked enough about the challenges to have made that clear. However, as we've also made clear: it's very much doable. That said, it's much easier to do when you're intrinsically motivated to succeed, or when your reasons for making those changes come from something you really want to do for yourself.

"It can be very easy to get discouraged as you make changes to your diet," says Elkrief. "That's why it's so important to be really in tune with those feelings of what you want and why you are doing this. What creates lasting, sustainable change is doing things because you really believe in it, feel connected to it, and find value in it. So, understanding why you want to make these changes—coming to terms with what anxiety or depression is taking from your life—is going to help you stay on track."

You want your motivations, whatever they may be, to outweigh any challenges you might face so that they can help you keep going even when you take a misstep. Because, as with any new endeavor, you're going to make mistakes from time to time.

Our goal is to help people find ways to make progress. Some people come to see us thinking they're going to overhaul their entire diet. That's just not realistic for most people. You take small steps, knowing there will be a learning curve as you go. You want your motivation to be strong enough that when you face challenges or make mistakes, you don't give up. Instead, you learn from that experience and keep on trying.

Be open to that learning process. When mistakes happen, it's not failure. It's a lesson. I could tell you many stories of all the mistakes I've made with food. When I first tried to add seafood to my own diet, needless to say there were many strangely seasoned and over-cooked pieces of fish. (There still are.) The first time I tried to make bacalao (salted codfish) fritters the fried fishy smell was so strong, I was transported back to my high school cafeteria. But those blunders came with both some important knowledge and some extra confidence. I discovered all the ways I do like to prepare seafood—and the ways my family will eat it. And, as I absorbed what *not* to do, I also became much more certain about where seafood fit into my weekly menu planning. I couldn't have done it without all the mess-ups to help guide me. You'll soon see that your mistakes are there to guide you, too.

SET GOALS FOR SUCCESS

As Elkrief says, eating to beat depression and anxiety isn't about overhauling your entire diet. That just isn't practical for most people. Rather, it's about making small, sustained changes that introduce more nutrient-dense foods from different categories into your dietary pattern so you can put your brain in a state of growth and plasticity. Remember, any journey starts with a single step. Similarly, learning how to change your diet happens bite by bite.

Management experts talk about SMART goals to help grow and maintain businesses. They'll tell you, as you set goals for yourself, that it's critical to make sure those goals are (s)pecific, (m)easurable, (a)chievable, (r)ealistic, and (t)imely.[1] It's no different when we're talking about eating habits. By going through all the steps of the self-assessment, you can better determine what your own SMART goals should be—and, in doing so, better set yourself up for success.

For example, maybe your assessment suggested you need to up your greens game. It also highlighted that you have some challenges around eating a healthy breakfast. You now have a great opportunity to know where to start. With that information in mind, during the leafy greens week of the six-week plan, maybe your goal will be to add your favorite green to your breakfast a few times during the course of a week. On Monday, you'll add greens to a smoothie using the Healthy-Brain Smoothie formula on page 224. Come Wednesday, you'll mix them into a tasty omelette or quiche. When Friday rolls around, you'll chop up your greens and add them to your favorite pasta. These goals are specific, measurable, achievable, realistic, and timely. They're ones you can easily set for yourself and meet. And, as you do so, you get the added benefit of building the knowledge, skills, and confidence you need to more successfully add greens to other meals.

After identifying opportunities for change, start out with goals that are small and specific. Then, when you achieve them, celebrate. When you're struggling with anxiety or depression, it's easy to discount the small wins. But make sure you acknowledge all the marks you're hitting so you can train your brain to see where you're succeeding—and continue to motivate yourself to make positive changes.

While food can be complicated, the way you eat to beat depression and anxiety doesn't have to be. You don't have to stop eating what you enjoy. You don't have to learn a whole new book's worth of brain-healthy recipes. You just have to determine where, when, and how you can add more nutrient-dense foods to the meals you already enjoy on a regular basis. Make your goals doable—and by adding up all your small wins, you'll soon see you've built a strong foundation that will lead to the kind of larger, lasting changes that can really bolster your mood and anxiety levels.

THE POWER LIES WITH YOU

Elkrief and I have learned that sustainable, healthy changes to a person's diet require more than just a list of foods and/or brain-healthy nutrients. It also requires taking a close look at an individual's relationship with food, dietary patterns, personal challenges, and motivation. Without that information, it's not only more difficult to generate the type of small, sustainable goals that can help you create a more joyful and nourishing connection with the foods you eat—but more challenging to develop the skills you'll need to translate small wins into bigger, long-term victories.

Remember, there's no one way to do this. No meal plan or strict protocol. This is about finding the self-awareness to really understand your habits—and extend some compassion to yourself as you work to feel better.

Some people may worry that six weeks isn't enough time. Others might try to make too many changes in a single week and then end up crashing. So, let me remind you, eater, that you have the power to heal yourself. Whatever way you approach the plan—and any missteps you may make along the way—are okay. You always have the opportunity to go back and try again. But, by taking the time to reflect on what shapes you as an eater—and the common challenges you face—you can put yourself in a stronger position to achieve these goals. You'll have the kind of self-awareness about your relationship with food that will make you feel more competent and confident, all while feeding your brain with the nutrients it needs to work its best. That's the kind of foundation you need to eat to beat depression and anxiety.

CHAPTER 7: Recap

- To ready yourself for Chapter 9's six-week plan, consider why you want to make changes to your dietary patterns. What are your primary concerns about your or a loved one's mental health?
- Take a look at your personal relationship with food. What was food like when you were growing up? Do you feel comfortable cooking? What are your go-to foods?
- Take the time to complete a food journal like the one in this chapter for a week to better understand your current dietary pattern. What do your typical meals look like? How and when do you snack? What are your strongest food emotions? How is your mood and anxiety?
- Before you start the plan, it's important to come up with SMART goals—or goals that are specific, measurable, achievable, realistic, and timely. What goals can you come up with each week that will enable you to rack up some small wins, setting you up for long-term success?
- Remember that, when it comes to diet, you have the power. There's no strict meal plan or protocol. But by taking the time to understand your background and habits, you're in a stronger position to embrace the next six weeks with competence and confidence.

· · · · · ·

Chapter 8

THE KITCHEN

Stock Up and Create the Ultimate Workspace to Feed Mental Health

Famed New York Yankee Yogi Berra once quipped, "Ninety percent of the game is half mental." He was referring to baseball, of course—but you can apply this same formula to setting and achieving most goals in life. In the last two chapters, you learned how to better prepare for the mental aspects of changing your dietary patterns. By considering the common challenges that today's eaters face, as well as doing your own personal food assessment, you've discovered what's been holding you back from adding more brain-healthy foods to your meals. You've also identified great places to start making some easy swaps or substitutions to add more nutrient-dense options.

The next part—setting up your kitchen as a positive, reliable workspace—is easy. Too often, we let the time it takes to buy and prepare food be a barrier to brain health. Or maybe we're intimidated by our lack of experience or skills in the kitchen. I can't tell you how many people I've met who've been convinced they can't cook have learned, with a little time and a little practice, that they, too, can become masters of self-nourishment. Simply put, having the right mind-set, coupled with some basic tools and pantry staples, puts you in a position to be more thoughtful and efficient when it comes time to planning and creating your meals. A big part of eating for mental health involves creating the kind of workspace that makes it easy to prepare your favorite foods from different food categories.

In this chapter, we'll highlight the tools, spices, and techniques that can help increase your kitchen efficiency and approach the six-week plan with confidence. Practicing your skills allows you to enjoy the kitchen without worry, so you can better sustain a lifestyle of nourishing your mental health over the long haul. It can also inspire you to try new foods and recipes as you build up your experience.

There are many good reasons why people don't eat for brain health. You likely discovered a few of your own as you filled out your food assessment. Maybe life is busy and you haven't felt like you've had enough time to cook. Perhaps you feel a little intimidated by putting together a dish. Maybe, because of where or how you live, it's more challenging to get hold of the fresh fruits and veggies you need. Costs are likely to be a consideration, too.

Trying to eat healthy on a budget can seem like more of a challenge than it actually is. Perhaps, because of your symptoms, you've simply lacked the motivation or energy to get started. No matter what your reasons might be, setting up the right space in your kitchen—tackling the physical part of Yogi Berra's success formula—can better support you as you start and then complete the six-week plan. Let's get started.

WHAT'S IN YOUR KITCHEN?

Before you do anything else, it pays to take stock of your current setup. Take a good look around your kitchen and take a mental inventory of what's in your cupboards and pantry. What kinds of foods do you have on hand? (For example, what are your go-to snacks and where are they located?) What might be hiding deep in the recesses of your freezer? Or, for that matter, in the doors of your fridge? What kind of utensils and appliances are in your drawers? What tools do you use on a regular basis? Which ones haven't seen the light of day in a while? What's your appliance situation? How are you storing food? Are there any herbs or spices lying around? Are they within easy reach of your stove?

The idea here is to figure out what you have to work with—and clean out what's no longer needed. While the idea of reorganizing your kitchen may seem as appealing as doing your taxes, it can be a great way to start building the workspace you need to inspire success. Those mystery meats in the back of your freezer? Chances are, they've gone bad and are taking vital space away from the frozen berries, greens, or seafood you could put there instead. Those chips or salty snacks taking up prime, easy-to-grab real estate in the cupboard? That sounds like a great spot to put nuts, seeds, and other brain-healthy snacks so they become your go-tos when you're feeling a little peckish. By taking a lay of the land, so to speak, you can figure out how to best reconfigure the kitchen to create the kind of functional efficiency that makes it easier to follow the six-week plan.

Don't let the idea of cleaning out your kitchen stress you out. You don't have to do it all at once—and it's not something you should worry yourself over. Rather, as you start the plan, maybe spend ten minutes a day doing a little cleanup. On day one, toss out all the old stuff in your freezer. Day two, go through your drawers, removing the clutter and consolidating your most important kitchen tools. Day three can be all about taking stock of your pantry. On day four, you can tackle organizing your spice rack. Within a week or two, you'll find you've done the work to optimize your workspace in a way to better help you eat for mental health.

Remember, every journey begins with a single step. Contrary to popular belief, you don't need a huge space or tons of gadgets to have a practical and useful kitchen. It's all about organizing what you do have so you can easily find what you need when you need it. Once you have a more functional space, you'll see that building a foundation to eat to beat depression and anxiety only involves the combination of a few basic tools, fresh ingredients, some tasty herbs and spices, and a simple willingness to add more nutrient-dense foods to your diet.

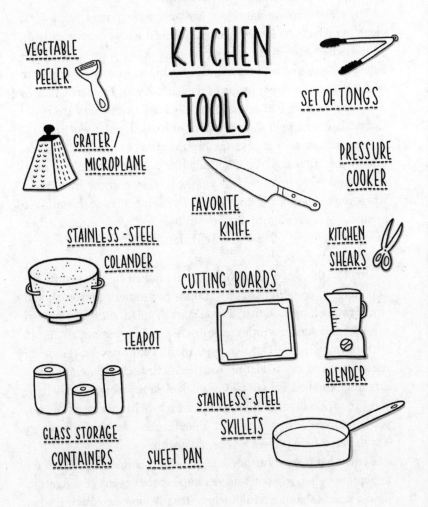

KITCHEN TOOLS

VEGETABLE PEELER

SET OF TONGS

GRATER / MICROPLANE

PRESSURE COOKER

FAVORITE KNIFE

STAINLESS-STEEL COLANDER

KITCHEN SHEARS

CUTTING BOARDS

TEAPOT

BLENDER

STAINLESS-STEEL SKILLETS

GLASS STORAGE CONTAINERS

SHEET PAN

BUILDING YOUR ESSENTIAL TOOLKIT

Having the right arsenal of kitchen tools to help you on your journey as you eat to beat depression and anxiety is easier than you might think. Below, I'll highlight some of the tools you can use to help master the recipes in the following chapter. You don't need to have all or even most of them to be successful. Your most basic toolkit only requires a good knife, a metal colander, a cutting board, a saucepan, a sauté pan, and a desire to eat more brain-healthy meals. That's it.

As you move forward and perhaps feel a little more ambitious, you might want to invest in some additional items in order to make more of the recipes outlined in the six-week plan.

Here are our recommended kitchen tools:

Tongs. Having cooking tongs on hand that easily open and close can assist in preparing everything from a basic salad to your favorite stir-fry. Grab tongs that are dishwasher-safe for easy cleanup so you can toss, turn, and grab your favorite foods from the oven, skillet, or grill.

Cutting Boards. It's hard to go wrong with cutting boards. Personally, I like the feel and look of wood, but plastic cutting boards are inexpensive, dishwasher-safe, and keep your countertops clean. Having a few boards on hand makes meal prep a breeze no matter what's on the menu. However, if you already have a trusty wood cutting board on hand, don't fret. It'll get the job done.

Vegetable Peeler. A good peeler does more than just shed the skins from your potatoes and carrots; it can also help you make your own zucchini noodles, peel fruits with tougher skins like citrus or mangoes, and shave cold butter or cheese. To help keep your peeler working its best, wash it by hand in warm water and soap to protect the blades.

Knives. You can find many kitchen knives with a range of different price points in most stores. The key is finding a knife you love for regular use and keeping it sharp. Find a sturdy paring knife or two, an 8-inch chef's knife, and a 10-inch serrated knife for bread. Having the right knives on hand helps you chop, mince, dice, and slice like a pro. To help your knives keep their edge longer, make sure to always wash them by hand.

Oyster Shucker. This special type of blade helps you free oysters and other shellfish from their shells. Look for one with a good grip so you can easily shuck your favorite filter feeder while keeping your hands safe.

Grater. Whether it's an old-fashioned box-handled cheese grater or a simple Microplane grater, graters help you grate everything from garlic to cheese to citrus zest. Most graters are dishwasher safe, which makes cleanup a breeze.

Stainless-Steel Colander. This is one of the most used items in my kitchen. A basic colander can help you do everything from wash your favorite fruits and veggies to strain pasta. Trust me—once you have one on hand, you'll wonder how you ever lived without it.

Kitchen Shears. A sharp pair of kitchen shears can help you cut everything from fresh herbs to chicken breasts. Look for a pair with stainless-steel blades that can be safely cleaned in your dishwasher. Some can even be taken apart for easier cleaning.

Blender. To make short work of chopping, dicing, or blending, having a blender with a high-power motor is a boon. While you can certainly find uses for mini blenders (for single servings), immersion blenders (to blend soups or smoothies directly in the pot or jar), or a food processor (the master of slicing, dicing, and shredding), larger blenders can take on many of those multiple duties. While high-end blenders like the Vitamix or Blendtec are pricey, lower-cost options are out there. Invest in the sturdiest, most powerful one you can afford to change the way you make soups, smoothies, pestos, and sauces.

Stainless-Steel Skillets. There are plenty of skillet sets available for purchase, but, for our purposes, you need only one large and one small stainless-steel skillet on hand to make your favorite sautéed, pan-fried, and braised meals. If you want to go the extra mile, pick up a cast-iron skillet to join the bunch. While cast-iron pans do require a little more work to season and clean, they can be used both on the stovetop and in the oven—and are great for vegetarians to get a little more iron in their diets.

Sheet Pan. Baking sheets aren't just for cookies anymore! A rimmed baking sheet will help you make the most of batch cooking or sheet meals each week—and is remarkably inexpensive. Going with a stainless-steel option makes for easy cleanup. You can just throw the pan in your dishwasher when you're done.

Slow Cooker, Rice Cooker, and Instant Pot. There's good reason why all your friends have gotten an Instant Pot over the past few years. This slow cooker on steroids can replace your traditional slow cooker, pressure cooker, rice cooker, steamer, and air-fryer. Just throw a few ingredients in and the Instant Pot will quickly and reliably do the rest. If you aren't jumping on the Instant Pot bandwagon, I heartily recommend having a rice cooker or slow cooker. They are two of my favorite tools. A rice cooker can cook your grains perfectly each and every time—and slow cookers are great for easy, one-pot slow-cooked meals like chicken vegetable soup or chili for a cold winter day.

Glass Storage Containers. While many people adore their Tupperware, I recommend the use of glass storage containers for a few reasons. First, it makes it very easy to see what's in your fridge or freezer. No mystery leftovers to puzzle out! But glass storage containers have additional benefits. They are more eco-friendly, hold heat better than plastic options, and don't leach unwanted chemicals into your food like plastic containers are apt to.

HEALTHY STAPLES AND STORES

Now that you have your tools squared away, it's time to consider your food stores. Most Americans have cupboards full of sugary, processed products. With those items on your shelves, there's no room for the nutrient-dense foods that will help you put your brain into grow mode. Consider replacing those junk foods with the following grains, legumes, and other fresh and frozen ingredients so you always have brain-boosting options within reach.

Grains

Sometimes, all you really want is a piece of toast—I get it!—but when you look beyond everyday baked goods, you'll find a wealth of different grains out there that can both jazz up your meals and offer a more diverse set of phytonutrients to your diet. By swapping out the typical refined white flour commonly used in basic white breads and pastas with more complex carbohydrates in whole grains, you'll quickly find that you can satisfy your carb cravings while getting more of the brain-boosting nutrients you need. Here are a few grains to have on hand:

Rice. There's a reason why so many cultures rely on this grass seed as a foundational ingredient. It's simple, versatile, and tasty. While you're likely more familiar with white rice, produced by "polishing" or removing the outer layer of the seed, brown, wild, and black varieties—which leave this outer layer intact—have more nutrient density, including that important brain-healthy B1 vitamin, thiamine. Use your Instant Pot or rice cooker and add this great grain to your greens, rainbow veggies, and salmon for an easy meal. And check out the Brainbow Kimchi Fried Rice on page 198.

Quinoa and Amaranth. Both of these pseudocereal grains have gained popularity over the past few years, for good reason. They were staples of the ancient Aztecs—and boast both high protein and monosaturated polyunsaturated fat content. They also contain a number of vitamins, minerals, and phytonutrients noted in the AFS. Added bonus? Both are quick and easy to prepare.

Steel-Cut Oatmeal. Oats have thoroughly earned the nickname "grain for the brain." This slow-burning carbohydrate is a great breakfast staple—and can give you a great energy boost. Steel-cut oats also contain important phytonutrients, as well as choline—the B-vitamin relative linked to a decrease in anxiety symptoms—that give them that little extra oomph. A word of caution: don't go for the easy instant variety oatmeal packets that take up the bulk of space on grocery shelves. Most of those are full of sugar. Instead, cook up a pot of steel-cut oats and then sweeten them yourself with honey, berries, or dark chocolate. You can also create savory oatmeal dishes. Try pairing oats with cheddar, chives, and a fried egg.

Millet. If you're looking for a grain with a ton of protein and fiber, millet tops the list. It's also an excellent source of magnesium and polyphenols. The foxtail variety of this grain even contains calcium! While millet is often overlooked in the United States, it is the sixth most consumed grain worldwide. Like rice, it's easy to add to greens or rainbows for an easy brain-healthy meal.

Beans and Legumes

One of the best—and most economical—ways to add more nutrient density to any meal is to include a handful of beans or legumes. Popular choices like chickpeas, lentils, and kidney beans offer eaters a unique plant-based protein with the added bonus of phyto-nutrients, minerals, and essential B vitamins. They're also an incredible value. You can grab a pound of dried beans at any grocery store for just a few dollars—and, in doing so, make sure you're getting a serious increase in the various nutrients that help your brain work its best.

Herbs

You can enhance the flavor of any meal with the well-placed addition of a few herbs. An added benefit of the fresh varieties is that they provide a little extra of the vital phytonutrients you want on top of the foods they season. While the recipes in the next chapter will make some suggestions on the best ways to pair different herbs with foods, it never hurts to experiment. Here are some ideas of how you can use herbs to create brain-boosting meals to titillate your taste buds.

Basil. There are several delicious varieties of basil—from Italian to sweet Thai. Try a few to find your favorite. Whichever you end up choosing, you'll soon see how well this herb pairs with veggies and fruits with a high-water content like tomatoes and zucchini—as well as some of your favorite cheeses. It also adds a nice zest to white fish, chicken, and shrimp. It's a great herb to play with as you add new food categories to your weekly meal plans.

Chives. You may not realize that chives are a special type of onion. That's one of the reasons they're such a versatile herb—they add an extra bite of flavor to fish or your favorite rainbow vegetables. They also add a little more zing to your favorite soups, sauces, and salad dressings. This is definitely a great one to have on hand for when you want to add just a little something extra.

Cilantro. Warning: to a certain percentage of people, cilantro tastes like soap. But the rest of us can appreciate its lemony, floral flavor when added to vegetables, chicken, and fish. If you're new to this herb, try it first cooked in a Mexican or Thai dish. It offers a mellower taste in a cooked preparation. Once you start to appreciate what cilantro adds to those dishes, feel free to explore by adding it to beans, potatoes, or mushrooms. Check out the Pesto Formula on page 188 using cilantro.

Parsley. You may have noticed that many of the meals you order in restaurants are garnished with fresh parsley. Why? It's available year-round and offers a fresh, springtime flavor. You can use parsley in your favorite soups and sauces and on meats and fish—it really is a "catchall" kind of herb.

Sage. This strong, savory herb is great for both grilling and marinades. It's also a tasty addition to a simple olive oil and garlic sauce for veggies and pasta. If you're new to this herb, given its pungency, it's best to start with a single leaf and build up from there. But, in time, I'm certain you'll be adding it to a variety of dishes, including butternut squash, potatoes, chicken, and your favorite pastas.

Rosemary. This herb is a great addition to meat marinades. Not only does it give a unique flavor to those dishes, it also adds some extra phytonutrients like rosmarinic acid and rosmanol, which have anti-inflammatory properties researched for their impressive neuroprotective attributes. Chop up a fresh sprig or two, or just add a pinch of a dried variety, to dress up some of your favorite meals.

Tarragon. You may be surprised to learn that tarragon is actually related to the bright, cheerful sunflower. This herb's licorice flavor is a mainstay of popular French dishes—and pairs well with everything from grapefruit to asparagus. One of my favorite ways to use tarragon is with a citrus zest to flavor grilled fish.

Thyme. Thyme is a member of the mint family. It's a common ingredient of soups, stews, roasts, and baked fish. It has a rather pungent taste—so a little goes a long way. But it's a welcome addition to help intensify the natural flavors found in popular herb mixes like herbes de Provence and Italian seasoning blends.

Spices

You may have heard that cooking a good dish is all about the right seasonings. As you find ways to work with more foods from the different categories, the addition of your favorite spices can help dishes go from "okay" to "wow." Here are a few of the different spices you should keep handy to not only add that extra bit of flavor, but also to add more vitamins and phytonutrients to your meals.

Black Pepper. Freshly ground pepper adds an earthy edge to anything. It's high in antioxidant molecules and also boasts anti-inflammatory properties.

Chiles. To add some heat to meats and veggies, chile flakes are great for perking up your meals. Chiles are chock-full of vitamin C, as well as potassium and vitamin B6, and add that little extra kick for those who like it hot. Salt-and-sugar-free chili powder (a blend of spices) is another option.

Cumin. This is a universal though often underutilized spice. From gumbo to chili to lentils to hummus, cumin adds a subtle punch to many popular foods. Its unique, earthy flavor not only warms up any dish but also provides some extra phytonutrients and an additional dose of iron.

Curry. This mix of spices is a mainstay of Indian cuisine and offers more than a unique, spicy flavor—it has also been shown to boost your immune system and keep your circulatory system in tip-top shape. You can use curry powder in a variety of different soups and stews, as well as to flavor veggies, fish, and chicken.

Garlic Powder. I've met more than a few people who have difficulty digesting the raw stuff, and sometimes you don't have the time or desire to mince garlic. No worries, as garlic powder offers the same flavor to your favorite dishes without the muss or fuss. Note: garlic salt is just garlic powder mixed with table salt. Make sure to adjust any recipe using garlic salt to make sure you don't overdo the sodium.

Turmeric. With a sour, pungent flavor that can add a little je ne sais quoi to both Eastern and Western dishes, turmeric is not only a spice but also an important player in Ayurvedic medicine. It's a flavor that works in both main dishes and desserts, provided you use it sparingly. To get an extra brain boost, pair turmeric with black pepper. It can increase the absorption of curcumin, one of the spice's active ingredients linked to increased BDNF expression.

Cooking Fats

Those who want to keep their car's engine running at top speed are usually willing to spend a little more on a higher-quality motor oil. The same analogy applies to the oils you use for cooking. Don't undo all the work you're doing to improve your diet by using fake or ultra-saturated fats in your meal prep. Instead, go for brain-healthy, organic monounsaturated fats. Buy smaller bottles and store them away from direct sunlight to prevent them from oxidizing. Also use the lowest heat possible when cooking with those fats to enhance nutrient absorption from your favorite rainbow veggies. While there are many different cooking fats available, I recommend sticking to three: olive oil, grass-fed butter, and coconut oil.

Olive Oil. It's said that what's good for the heart is good for the brain—and olive oil, which contains a special phytonutrient called hydroxytyrosol, protects your blood vessels to keep both your cardiovascular and nervous systems in top working order. There's a reason why health experts agree this should be a part of any healthy diet. Olive oil is also a cornerstone of the Mediterranean diet and has not only been shown to help prevent and manage depressive symptoms but also to fight inflammation.

Grab a bottle of extra-virgin olive oil (EVOO), which has more of the phytonutrients you seek. If you have recipes that require higher heat, grab a refined olive oil with a higher smoke point.

Grass-Fed Butter. Leave the margarine or other whipped vegetable oil spreads on the grocery shelf. Grass-fed butter not only offers a richer, creamier flavor but also has the healthy fats that assist in building muscle and brain cells. In addition, grass-fed butter contains other vitamins and minerals that play a vital role in brain development and maintenance. If you're looking to be a little adventurous, you can also try ghee, the clarified butter used in traditional Indian recipes. It has a higher smoke point than butter and a lovely nutty flavor that brings that little something extra to fish or veggie dishes.

Coconut Oil. This oil is also free of undesired trans fats and is a great option for your favorite stir-fries. While its status as a superfood remains controversial, coconut oil has been shown to have some anti-inflammatory properties and is comprised of medium-chain triglycerides (MCTs). These fats are being researched to help with brain energy consumption in Alzheimer's disease and are used by people eating keto to help them stay in ketosis.

Frozen Foods

While fresh, in-season fruits, vegetables, and proteins are generally your best bet for getting the most phytonutrients per bite, we understand that buying fresh isn't always possible. There are still a lot of nutrients to be found in frozen options and they're available year-round in your grocery's freezer section. In order to easily put together a brain-boosting breakfast smoothie or stir-fry, just reach into your freezer and go.

Berries and Fruits. Looking for an easy breakfast? Frozen blueberries, strawberries, and peaches are there for the taking. Sometimes you can even find more exotic fruits like mangoes and pomegranates. In the morning, just grab a handful of your frozen fruit of choice and add it to your smoothie like you would any fresh variety. It will give you a taste of summer all year round.

Greens. Spinach, broccoli, kale, and brussels sprouts also freeze well. Have frozen varieties on hand to quickly add to stir-fries, slow-cooker dishes, or sheet-pan meals.

Seafood. Not all of us have a local fishmonger to visit for the day's fresh catch. But many types of seafood freeze quite well. Sea bass, salmon, and shrimp are all easy to keep in your freezer for nights when you're craving a good meal.

These aren't the only types of frozen foods that can help in your quest to eat to beat depression; you likely already have some chicken or beef in your freezer. But by thinking outside the old-fashioned, TV dinner–type frozen meal, you can easily ensure that you always have healthy, nutrient-dense options on hand when it comes time to eat.

SHOPPING TIPS

The grocery store is full of all kinds of temptations. If you do your shopping by walking up and down the aisles, chances are you'll end up picking up a lot of foods you don't really need—especially more of the saltier, sugary processed foods that you're better off avoiding. To help make sure you have the right ingredients on hand to eat to beat depression and anxiety, try to stick to the perimeter of the store. That's where you'll find fresh fruits, veggies, seafood, meats, and other items for the six-week plan. Then make a quick swing by the grain and frozen foods sections to pick up any other items you may need.

PLANNING AHEAD

When you aren't feeling your best, the idea of making dinner—or any other meal, for that matter—may seem overwhelming. Sometimes it makes me feel that way even when I'm not feeling down! That's why planning ahead is important. By using batch-cooking techniques, where you prepare several meals ahead of time, you can make sure you always have a few days' worth of breakfasts, lunches, and dinners available for when you aren't up to cooking.

Similarly, if you find the prospect of cleanup daunting, sheet-pan meals may be the way to go. All you need to do is throw some healthy ingredients on a single sheet pan and put it in the oven. There are all manner of recipes available that will ensure that you'll never be bored with what you cook. But the best part is that, once it's done, all you need to do is wash a knife or two and your baking sheet. Slow cookers and Instant Pots are also great when it comes to "throw and go" type meals with easier cleanup.

Planning ahead also makes it much easier to appropriately portion things out. Too often, especially when we're struggling with mental health, we eat too much or too little. By taking the time to divide up what you cook into individual portions, you can better ensure that you and your family are getting exactly what you really need.

DON'T BE AFRAID OF SHORTCUTS

As I said before, the goal of this chapter is to highlight the different tools and techniques that can help increase your efficiency in the kitchen—setting you up for success as you start Chapter 9's six-week plan. Though there are many reasons why people don't eat for optimal brain health, by taking the time to prepare—both mentally and physically—you can get to a place where you can make the most of the six-week plan. Before you know it, you'll be on your own path to consistently nourishing your mental health.

However, if you aren't as experienced in the kitchen or have been struggling with your mental health, I can understand if you find some of this prep work a little daunting. That's why I want to emphasize the most important canon of all: it's not cheating to take a few shortcuts. You don't need to have a fully kitted and stocked kitchen to eat to beat depression and anxiety. The only essential ingredient is your willingness to make a few changes to your diet. If you aren't up for trying a new recipe yet, think about ways you can add a food or two from the different categories to your favorite dishes. Identify a few places where you can make easy switches or swaps.

Maybe the idea of shopping is a little too much right now. There's no reason why you can't use one of the many different meal-prep kits available in your grocery's deli section—or even sign up for one of the popular ingredient and recipe meal kit services. If that's the best way for you to add leafy greens, rainbow veggies, and seafood to your weekly meals, then no harm, no foul.

And if you don't want to cook at all? That works, too. There's no reason why you can't get the nutrients you need from your favorite takeout joints. Ask your restaurants of choice if they can add some extra spinach or arugula to your favorite dish. Go a little out of your comfort zone and order the daily fish special or a spicy vegetable stir-fry. Use the knowledge you've learned about the AFS and the food categories to select items that can help you increase your meals' nutrient density.

As I've said before, eating to beat depression and anxiety happens bite by bite. How you get to that first bite is entirely up to you. There's no reason to feel shame or guilt about what strategies help you get there.

Just as I tell my patients that I don't judge what or how they eat, you shouldn't judge your progress, either. Your unique tastes, values, and approaches to eating are yours alone. If your personal tactics are helping you work toward changing those old, ingrained habits to include more nutrient-dense foods in your meals, you're already ahead of the game. What I often see is that, as patients improve their diet quality and start feeling better, they're willing to be a little more adventurous in the kitchen. Eventually they gain the confidence and the know-how to better shop and prepare foods for themselves. It doesn't have to be gourmet to get the job done.

In the next chapter, we'll go over the six-week plan step-by-step, addressing the areas we've seen are the most beneficial to eaters as they change their dietary patterns. If you've worked through your food assessment and looked at kitchen space and stores, you've already done the hard part. You've set yourself up for success. Now it's time to go over the game plan and begin your journey to becoming a master of self-nourishment. Let's get to it.

CHAPTER 8: Recap

- Setting up your kitchen is another important part of eating to beat depression and anxiety. It gives you the ability to be more thoughtful and efficient when it comes time to plan and create your meals.
- Take time to take stock of your current kitchen. What tools do you have? What basic stores of food do you always have on hand? What clutter might be getting in the way?
- The most basic kitchen toolkit only requires a good knife, a metal colander, a cutting board, a saucepan, a sauté pan, and a desire to eat more brain-healthy meals. As you gain more confidence, you may want to invest in other kitchen items, like tongs, a vegetable peeler, a grater, an oyster shucker, a pair of kitchen shears, and glass storage containers.
- Having a pantry stocked with stores of legumes and grains can help ensure you always have a healthy addition for soups and salads within reach. Having herbs and spices to add flavor to your favorite brain-healthy dishes is also a boon.

- Planning ahead can be a great advantage, especially if you're trying to eat to beat depression and anxiety when you aren't feeling your best. By making batch meals one or two days a week, you can be sure you always have a nutrient-dense option available come mealtime.
- Don't be afraid of shortcuts! You don't need a fully stocked kitchen to find success. Instead of trying to overhaul your entire cooking workspace, start with some easy switches and swaps.

Chapter 9

. . . .

THE SIX-WEEK PLAN
AND RECIPES

You've learned a lot about how food impacts your brain health, as well as the specific foods and food categories that can help you eat to beat depression and anxiety. It's now time to put that knowledge into action. The six-week plan is a jumping-off point I created to help people who are struggling with mood or anxiety symptoms—but just don't quite know where to begin. I use plans like this one all the time at the Brain Food Clinic. It's a great way to help my patients find a simple, personalized, and sustainable way to change their diet to include more brain-healthy nutrients.[1]

I'm not asking you to overhaul your entire diet. That's just not realistic. I'm also not here to force you to eat foods you don't like; that won't help in the long run, either. Rather, this six-week plan will provide simple guidance, one week at a time, to highlight the common areas where Samantha Elkrief and I have seen our patients find the most success. Our goal is to equip you with a strong foundation for brain-healthy eating that you can build upon over time. How you eat to beat depression and anxiety today will likely not look the same as it does six weeks, three months, or even a year from now. As you try new dishes, improve your kitchen skills, and gain more confidence in how to best nourish your brain, you'll find your dietary patterns slowly but surely evolving. That's the way to do it.

Each week's section will address a specific food category and include information about goals, easy swaps and substitutions, challenges, and simple, delicious recipes. At the end of each week, there's an assessment to help celebrate your successes as you achieve your unique SMART goals—those specific, measurable, achievable, realistic, and timely objectives you put into place. It's also a place where you can consider where things maybe didn't go as well as planned, so you can identify what you might tweak next time.

Over the next six weeks, you'll notice how each food category builds on the other; foods from the previous week are integrated into the subsequent week's recipes and meal planning. Then, once these four critical food categories are in place, the plan adds in foods that can help support a healthy, diverse microbiome. Finally, during the last week of the plan, we ask you to think about your food roots and how a better connection to your food culture, local food system, and greater food community can help you continue to best nourish your brain long after you finish the six weeks.

Treat it like your new mantra: there's no one single way to eat to beat depression and anxiety. While we've included recipes for you to try, they're not part of any requisite meal plan. They're jumping-off points for integrating more nutrient-dense foods into your diet, but they're certainly not the only way to do so. As you move through the next six weeks, figure out what works for you. Instead of cooking up a green shakshuka for breakfast, maybe you feel more comfortable adding a handful of kale or watercress to your scrambled eggs. Perhaps you still feel a little intimidated about cooking your own seafood dishes at home, but, like Pete, you're open to ordering some fish tacos from your favorite takeout joint. There are many roads to success. The only requirement is that you get on one of them. I assure you, no matter your current dietary pattern or specific eating challenges, there *is* a path forward for you.

Your greatest asset is your brain. You want to keep it as healthy as possible for both yourself and those you love. By using this evidence-based plan as a starting point, you can develop the skills and expertise to eat to beat depression and anxiety—and support brain health for a lifetime.

One note before we get started: while the following plan is designed to occur over a six-week period, with each lesson building on the one before it, there's no reason why it can't be an eight-, twelve-, or even thirty-week plan. Making changes to your diet can be challenging, especially if you're struggling with your mental health. The goal is progress, not perfection—and everyone has their own pace. If you didn't meet your goals one week, or if you weren't feeling up to continuing another week, that's okay. You can always redo a food category to help you better meet your goals. In fact, if you need to, you can repeat a category several times to get to where you want to be. If you had to take some time away from the plan for a week or two, just pick up where you left off. Life happens. Don't let guilt or shame get in the way of building your skills to better nourish your brain. How you eat to beat depression and anxiety is entirely up to you. If you need more time to get there, I promise it won't diminish your ultimate success.

WEEK 1: LEAFY GREENS (AND OTHER COLORS)

There's a reason why everyone—no matter what kind of diet they may be recommending—is on board with leafy greens. Kale, mustard greens, spinach, and watercress are the foundation of the Earth's food supply. When you track how almost any food you love comes into existence, you'll likely see it all started with an energy source and a leaf. That's one of the biggest reasons why leafy greens (or reds or purples—we don't discriminate) should be included in most of the meals you eat.

When you include an ample serving of leaves in your diet, you can ensure you're getting more hydration, satiation, and nutrient density with every meal. You're also getting that vital fiber that your microbiome loves, as well as a myriad of phytonutrients, vitamins, and minerals to keep your body and brain in top shape.

Consider a simple cup of kale. It contains only 33 calories but gives you over 600% of your daily recommended vitamin K, 200% of your daily vitamin A, and 134% of your vitamin C, not to mention iron, folate, calcium, and its array of inflammation-fighting phytonutrients. That's a whole lot of nutrition.

During this week, the goal is to try to eat at least **1 to 2 packed cups of chopped greens** per day—more if you can manage it. (If this seems like a lot, a quick sauté or wilt in soup for sauce reduces this amount to a few bites. For an example see the Turkey Zucchini Skillet Lasagna on page 200.)

How to Start

Look back over the food assessment you completed in Chapter 7. Where are you when it comes to greens? Is your greens game already on point, getting those 1 to 2 cups each day? If so, perhaps your goal this week should be to vary them. Try some sunflower seed sprouts or mustard greens instead of your usual go-to varieties.

If greens are a challenge for you, one of the easiest ways to start adding these nutrient powerhouses into your diet is by blending up a brain-boosting smoothie. Throw half a banana, some berries, a handful of walnuts, a cup of kale, and some ice and kefir into the blender for a tasty, filling breakfast that will truly up the brain-nutrient ante for you. You can also lean on your favorite foods as a vehicle for these greens. Many of my patients throw watercress into cheesy scrambled eggs or add extra spinach to a lasagna or enchiladas. When you think about your SMART goals for this week, identify easy swaps, substitutions, or enhancements to your go-to meals to get that cup of this nutrient-dense food.

Tips and Tricks

One of my favorite things about leaves is their amazing versatility. When you ask people about greens, the first thing many mention is an iceberg lettuce salad. Boring! There are so many other amazing ways to add greens to your meals. The salad is a great place to start, of course. Susan, for example, got a lot of mileage from swapping out iceberg lettuce for arugula and red-leaf lettuce. You, too, can increase the quality of your salad by adding in your favorite leafy green. But you can also grind greens into a tasty pesto, add some to your go-to sauté, or fold them into a flavorful stir-fry. Leaves are truly a category where you're limited only by your imagination.

I'm often asked whether we should be eating our greens raw or cooked. And my answer is always a resounding yes! Eat them both ways. If you simmer down your greens, it's true that you'll lose some of the folate and heat-sensitive phytonutrients. Regardless, you'll still get a massive dose of healthy vitamins and minerals in each and every bite. And if you're feeling a bit reticent about eating raw greens, you should know that the right dressing or sauce—like the rich, creamy, garlic-based dressing in the All Kale Caesar (page 180)—really makes all the difference.

This is a wonderful time to explore. Most supermarkets boast a cornucopia of fresh, mixed, frozen, and bagged options that make it easy to add this food to any meal. Truly, when you start to think outside the salad, you'll soon see that greens can be a core component of breakfast, lunch, or dinner. You can start your day with a mouthwatering green shakshuka for breakfast, followed by a simmering bowl of caldo verde for lunch, and then top it all off with your favorite dish paired with pesto for dinner. Delicious!

Challenge

The biggest challenge for most people is finding new ways to eat greens. But once they try new dishes and different styles of preparation, they discover how much they enjoy eating leaves—certainly more than they thought they would. One note, however: unwashed leafy greens are a common vector for pathogens like *E. coli*, salmonella, and listeria. Be sure to carefully wash them to avoid illness—just fill a bowl with cool water and swish the greens inside. All the dirt will accumulate at the bottom. Alternatively, you can buy bags of triple-washed leaves from the grocery store.

LEAFY GREENS

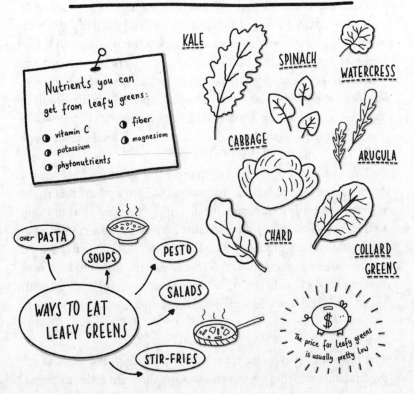

Green Shakshuka

SERVES 4

This dish delivers ample choline and B vitamins—key for stable moods and a calm mind. Start the day with eggs and greens? Yes, please! Make this year-round using any leafy green that you love . . . collards in the wintertime, Swiss chard and kale in the spring, and spinach in the summer, or use a combination. Serving this dish with crusty bread or pita is a fabulous way to scoop up all of the saucy greens and egg yolk, but the crunchy seeds provide a great texture and bite without the bread. To make a traditional tomato-based shakshuka but still get tons of greens in, use one 14.5-ounce can of diced tomatoes instead of the vegetable broth. Simmer until thickened to the consistency of a marinara sauce, then season to taste. Crack the eggs into this mixture.

2 tablespoons olive oil

2 large bunches Swiss chard (about 1½ pounds), stems and leaves coarsely chopped and kept separate (about 9 packed cups)

1 medium yellow onion, diced

3 garlic cloves, minced

1 teaspoon ground cumin

Kosher salt

½ teaspoon smoked paprika

¼ teaspoon red pepper flakes

¼ teaspoon ground turmeric

⅓ cup low-sodium vegetable broth

8 large eggs

3 ounces feta cheese, crumbled (about ¾ cup)

2 tablespoons chopped fresh cilantro

2 tablespoons chopped pepitas (pumpkin seeds)

Warm the olive oil in a 12-inch skillet over medium-high heat. Add the Swiss chard *stems only* and onion. Cook, stirring often, for 4 to 5 minutes, until tender.

Add the garlic, cumin, ¾ teaspoon salt, the paprika, red pepper flakes, and turmeric and cook, stirring, for 1 more minute, or until very fragrant. Stir in the Swiss chard leaves and vegetable broth and cook for 2 to 3 minutes, until the leaves are tender and most of the broth has evaporated.

Reduce the heat to medium-low. Using the back of a wooden spoon, create eight divots in the chard mixture. Crack an egg into each. Season the eggs with a pinch of salt. Cook until the whites are almost set, 5 to 7 minutes. Sprinkle the cheese over the top, then cover and cook until the whites are set and the yolks are cooked to your liking, 2 to 4 minutes more.

Serve in shallow bowls garnished with the cilantro and pepitas.

NUTRITIONAL STATS PER SERVING: 348 Calories, 21g Protein, 17g Carbohydrates, 22g Fat (7g Saturated), 369mg Cholesterol, 6g Sugars, 5g Fiber, 744mg Sodium

TOP NUTRIENTS: Vitamin A = 130%, Vitamin B12 = 125%, Vitamin C = 80%, Choline = 69%, Magnesium = 57%

All Kale Caesar

SERVES 4

This is my favorite way to eat kale and the basis of my best kale joke.* While any kale will work, the long, dark leaves of lacinato kale are best. This filling, rich salad features top power players of kale, anchovies, and cashews. The more anchovies, the more brain benefits, as each anchovy has 85 milligrams of long-chain omega-3 fats. Traditional Caesar dressings use raw egg; we swapped in soaked cashews for a little plant-based creaminess. And there is a crunch in every single bite with nutrient-dense Pepita-Parmesan Crunch instead of croutons!

Cashew-Caesar Dressing

4 oil-packed anchovies, drained

¼ cup (packed) grated Parmesan cheese

2 tablespoons raw cashews, preferably soaked in water overnight

3 Brazil nuts

1 large egg yolk, at room temperature

Juice of 1 large lemon (about 3 tablespoons)

1 teaspoon Dijon mustard

½ teaspoon garlic powder

½ cup olive oil

Kosher salt

Pepita-Parmesan Crunch

1½ tablespoons olive oil

½ cup panko breadcrumbs

½ cup finely chopped pepitas (pumpkin seeds)

2 tablespoons hemp hearts

¼ cup grated Parmesan cheese

¼ teaspoon garlic powder

⅛ teaspoon kosher salt

Salad

2 large bunches lacinato kale (about 1½ pounds)

¼ teaspoon kosher salt

To make the Cashew-Caesar Dressing:

Put the anchovies, cheese, cashews, Brazil nuts, egg yolk, lemon juice, mustard, and garlic powder in a blender and blend to combine. It might not get totally smooth—that's okay. With the motor running on low speed, very slowly pour in the olive oil and blend until emulsified. This should take about 1 minute total. Taste and season with salt as needed. The dressing should be about the consistency of mayonnaise; if needed, thin it out with 1 teaspoon of water at a time.

To make the Pepita-Parmesan Crunch:

Warm the olive oil in a large skillet over medium heat. Add the panko, pepitas, and hemp hearts and stir to coat in the oil. Toast, stirring often, for 4 to 5 minutes, until golden brown. Stir in the cheese, garlic powder, and salt and stir until the cheese melts and clings to the breadcrumbs and is nicely toasted, 15 to 20 seconds. Remove from the heat and allow to cool completely.

To make the salad:

Remove the ribs from the kale leaves, stack the leaves in a pile, and roll them up like a burrito. Then slice the leaves as thinly as possible. (This French slicing technique is called *chiffonade*.) Place the kale in a large bowl and sprinkle with the salt. Use both hands to massage the kale for about 10 seconds, until it feels slightly damp.

Toss in the desired amount of dressing to coat the kale. Sprinkle the Pepita-Parmesan Crunch over the top. Enjoy immediately.

While people think kale is a fad food, did you know kale was actually consumed in ancient Rome?! After all, they greeted each other, "All kale Caesar."

NUTRITIONAL STATS PER SERVING: 549 Calories, 16g Protein, 29g Carbohydrates, 41g Fat (7.5g Saturated), 60mg Cholesterol, 1g Sugar, 5g Fiber, 690mg Sodium

TOP NUTRIENTS: Vitamin C = 281%, Vitamin A = 194%, Selenium = 106%, Iron = 28%, Vitamin B12 = 21%

Brain-Food Salad

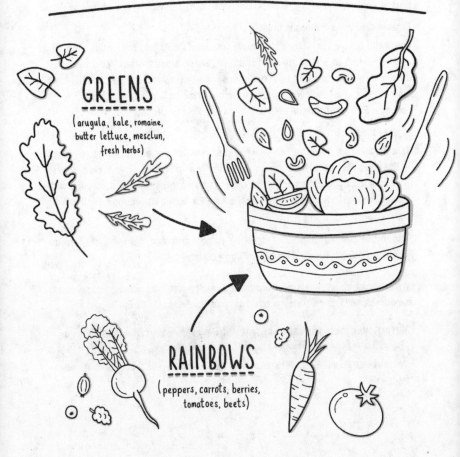

GREENS

(arugula, kale, romaine, butter lettuce, mesclun, fresh herbs)

RAINBOWS

(peppers, carrots, berries, tomatoes, beets)

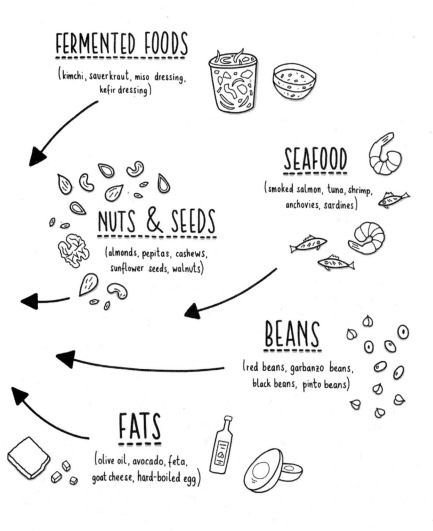

FERMENTED FOODS
(kimchi, sauerkraut, miso dressing,
kefir dressing)

SEAFOOD
(smoked salmon, tuna, shrimp,
anchovies, sardines)

NUTS & SEEDS
(almonds, pepitas, cashews,
sunflower seeds, walnuts)

BEANS
(red beans, garbanzo beans,
black beans, pinto beans)

FATS
(olive oil, avocado, feta,
goat cheese, hard-boiled egg)

Brain Food Cobb Salad

SERVES 4

This salad is as nutritious as it is gorgeous. It's bursting with citrus, avocado, and two excellent sources of protein: salmon and eggs. No need to worry about which came first—your brain gets both.

Serve on whole romaine leaves (fork and knife required) or, to make it easier to eat, thinly slice the romaine before assembling. Wild salmon takes this Cobb salad to the next level, as does a variation with seafood. You can also swap in grilled chicken or wild shrimp. Check out the Brain-Food Salad formula (page 182) for even more options.

Citrus Vinaigrette

- 1/3 cup grapefruit juice (from 1 medium grapefruit)
- 1/4 cup orange juice (from 1 large orange)
- 3 tablespoons fresh lemon juice (from 1 large lemon)
- 2 tablespoons Dijon mustard
- 2 tablespoons minced shallot
- 1/2 teaspoon kosher salt, plus more as needed
- 1/3 cup extra-virgin olive oil

Salad

- 8 ounces romaine lettuce, leaves separated
- Kosher salt and freshly ground black pepper
- 1 large orange, peeled and sliced into thin rounds
- 1 large grapefruit, peeled and sliced into thin rounds
- 1 large avocado, cubed
- 2 hard-boiled eggs, peeled and chopped
- 8 ounces cherry tomatoes, quartered
- 4 (6-ounce) wild salmon fillets, cooked
- 1/3 cup raw cashews, chopped
- 1/3 cup finely chopped fresh parsley leaves

To make the citrus vinaigrette:

Whisk the grapefruit juice, orange juice, lemon juice, mustard, shallot, and salt together in a large bowl. Whisking constantly, slowly pour in the olive oil until the dressing emulsifies. Taste and season with additional salt if needed.

To make the salad:

Arrange the romaine leaves across the bottom of a large shallow platter or bowl. Season with salt and pepper. Arrange the orange, grapefruit, avocado, hard-boiled eggs, and cherry tomatoes over the leaves in sections so that everyone can pick out their preferred amount of each ingredient. Arrange the salmon fillets over the top and scatter the cashews and parsley over everything.

Serve the citrus vinaigrette on the side.

NUTRITIONAL STATS PER SERVING: 578 Calories, 50g Protein, 27g Carbohydrates, 30g Fat (4.5g Saturated), 203mg Cholesterol, 15g Sugars, 8g Fiber, 510mg Sodium

TOP NUTRIENTS: Vitamin C = 128%, Vitamin B6 = 120%, Folate = 50%, Vitamin A = 43%, Potassium = 40%, Omega-3s (DHA+EPA) = 513% (2566mg)

Kale and Basil Pesto

SERVES 4

Pesto expands your greens intake beyond salads, stir-fries, and sautés. Use the formula to find your favorite combination. Basil and pine nuts are the classic pesto base, but there are so many other nuts and greens that make nutritious options. On our farm we started with this version by adding 1 cup of kale and swapping the pine nuts for cashews and pepitas, which deliver more iron and magnesium. For optimal freshness, and to avoid excess salt and added fats, use raw, unsalted nuts and seeds. You can deepen the flavor by toasting then cooling the nuts before adding them to the pesto. Place them on a baking sheet in a 350°F oven for 7 to 10 minutes, checking and tossing regularly, until browned.

We make and freeze pesto, as it is such a versatile base. For a killer creamy sauce great with grilled vegetables and meats, swap in 1/2 cup plain, whole-fat yogurt or sour cream for the olive oil. Or make it vegan by swapping in 1/3 cup nutritional yeast or miso for the Parmesan.

Kale Pesto

2 large lacinato kale leaves (about 1 cup)

Kosher salt

2 cups fresh basil leaves

1/2 cup grated Parmesan cheese

1/4 cup extra-virgin olive oil

1/4 cup unsalted, raw cashews (or try toasted—see headnote)

1/4 cup unsalted, raw pepitas (pumpkin seeds—see headnote)

2 Brazil nuts

2 garlic cloves, smashed and peeled

Juice of 1 large lemon (about 3 tablespoons), plus more as needed

1/2 teaspoon kosher salt

Pesto

Ingredients

- 3 cups fresh herbs or greens
- ½ cup grated parmesan cheese
- ¼ cup extra-virgin olive oil
- ¼ cup nuts
- 2 garlic cloves
- 1-2 teaspoons of acid
- ½ teaspoon kosher salt

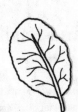
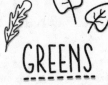

GREENS

(arugula, kale, swiss chard,
dandelion greens, beet greens, spinach,
basil, cilantro, parsley)

① Add all ingredients to a
blender and blend until smooth.

② Taste and season with more
salt and acid if needed.

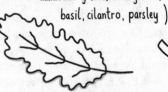

ACID

(lemon juice, lime juice,
any light-colored vinegar)

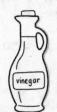

vinegar

FAT

(extra - virgin olive oil, avocado oil,
mayonnaise, sour cream, Greek yogurt)

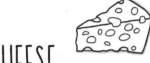

CHEESE

(Parmesan, Asiago, Pecorino Romano,
aged Cheddar or Gouda, Manchego

<u>dairy - free</u>: nutritional yeast, 2 tbsp miso,
⅓ cup coconut cream)

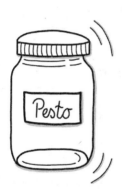

Pesto

NUTS & SEEDS

(cashews, walnuts, almonds, pine nuts, peanuts,
pumpkin / sesame / sunflower seeds,
macadamia nuts, pecans,
pistachios)

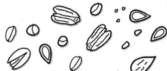

Remove the tough ribs from the kale leaves and discard them. Roughly chop the kale, sprinkle with salt, and use your hands to massage the leaves until they feel wet and soft, 15 to 20 seconds. Place in a food processor or blender.

Add the remaining ingredients and process until smooth. You may have to scrape down the sides a couple times. Taste and season with more salt and lemon juice if needed.

NUTRITIONAL STATS PER SERVING: 153 Calories, 6g Protein, 9g Carbohydrates, 10.5g Fat (3.1g Saturated), 10mg Cholesterol, 1g Sugar, 2g Fiber, 473mg Sodium

TOP NUTRIENTS: Selenium = 149%, Vitamin C = 36%, Vitamin A = 28%, Zinc = 13%, Magnesium = 7%

Pesto Formula

SERVES 4 (ABOUT 2 CUPS PESTO)

Each time I think I know pesto, I hear about an option I'd never considered: pistachios and sunflower seeds or cilantro and radicchio. That is part of pesto's role in fighting for your mental health—the endless variations and tastes. Use this formula to help you find your combinations.

3 cups fresh basil and greens
½ cup grated Parmesan cheese
¼ cup extra-virgin olive oil
¼ cup unsalted nuts (toasted or raw)
2 garlic cloves, smashed and peeled

1 to 2 tablespoons acid (lemon or lime juice, or a light-colored vinegar), plus more as needed
½ teaspoon kosher salt, plus more as needed

Combine all the ingredients in a food processor or blender and process until smooth, scraping down the sides as needed. Taste and season with more salt and acid if needed.

Caldo Verde

This classic, simple soup is very soothing and filling. Boosting soups with chopped greens is a simple move that adds to the versatility and accessibility of greens. You can also use collards, Swiss chard, or roughly chopped spinach. Chickpeas add fiber, protein, and iron. Look for a sausage with no preservatives, ideally from pasture-raised animals. No immersion blender? Use a slotted spoon to transfer the potatoes, chickpeas, and 2 cups of broth to a blender and mix until smooth. Be sure to allow it to cool slightly before blending to avoid an explosion!

- 2 tablespoons olive oil
- 1 medium yellow onion, roughly chopped
- 6 garlic cloves, roughly chopped
- 5 cups low-sodium chicken broth
- 8 ounces Yukon Gold potatoes, diced into 1-inch pieces
- 1 (15-ounce) can chickpeas, drained
- 1 bay leaf
- Kosher salt
- 1 large bunch kale (about 1 pound), ribs removed, thinly sliced
- 12 ounces precooked mild Italian chicken sausage, sliced 1/4-inch thick on a slight bias
- Juice of 1 large lemon (about 3 tablespoons)
- Freshly ground black pepper

Warm the olive oil in a large heavy-bottomed pot over medium-high heat. Add the onion and cook for 5 to 7 minutes, until softened. Add the garlic and cook for an additional 1 minute.

Stir in the chicken broth, potatoes, chickpeas, bay leaf, and 1 1/2 teaspoons salt. Bring to a boil over high heat, then reduce the heat to medium-low, cover, and cook for 20 minutes, or until the potatoes are fork-tender.

Remove the bay leaf, then use an immersion blender to blend the soup until smooth.

Raise the heat to medium, then stir in the kale and chicken sausage and continue cooking for 3 to 5 minutes, until the kale is wilted but still slightly crunchy.

Remove from heat. Stir in the lemon juice and season with salt and pepper.

NUTRITIONAL STATS PER SERVING: 436 Calories, 27.5g Protein, 43g Carbohydrates, 19g Fat (4g Saturated), 70mg Cholesterol, 3g Sugars, 9g Fiber, 827mg Sodium

TOP NUTRIENTS: Vitamin C = 207%, Vitamin A = 126%, Vitamin B6 = 46%, Iron = 50%, Potassium 20%, Zinc = 11%

Herby Prosciutto Chicken with Sautéed Greens

SERVES 4

Goodbye boring greens, hello chicken saltimbocca. This version of the classic Italian dish skips the flour and relies on prosciutto to add rich flavor and a crispy bite. Mix and match your choice of greens—Swiss chard, kale, beet greens, spinach, and bok choy are all great options for this delicious, quick-cooking side. Chicken breasts vary in size and weight. Two larger breasts can be cut in half lengthwise to form four 6-ounce pieces, if needed. To save time you can ask your butcher to cut and/or pound the breasts.

5 garlic cloves, divided

1 large lemon

¼ cup fresh parsley leaves, minced

¼ cup fresh basil leaves, minced

Kosher salt

¼ teaspoon freshly ground black pepper

2 tablespoons extra-virgin olive oil, divided, plus more as needed

4 (6-ounce) skinless, boneless chicken breasts, gently pounded to ⅓-inch thickness

4 slices prosciutto (about 3 ounces)

2 bunches Swiss chard (about 1¼ pounds), stems trimmed and thinly sliced, leaves roughly chopped (about 10 cups)

Using a Microplane or the smallest holes on a box grater, grate 3 of the garlic cloves and the zest of the lemon into a bowl. Stir in the parsley, basil, 1 teaspoon salt, the pepper, and 1 tablespoon of the olive oil.

Thinly slice the remaining 2 garlic cloves, cut the lemon in half, and set aside.

Rub the herb mixture all over the chicken. Place 1 slice of prosciutto over the smooth side of each breast, pressing to help it adhere.

Heat the remaining 1 tablespoon of oil in a large skillet over medium-high heat. Add the chicken, prosciutto-side down, in batches if necessary, and cook until the prosciutto side is crispy, 4 to 5 minutes. Turn the chicken and cook until the chicken is cooked through, about 3 minutes more.

Transfer the chicken to serving plates. Keep the skillet on medium-high heat. Add more oil if needed to reach 1 tablespoon in the skillet, then stir in the sliced garlic and half of the Swiss chard. Cook, stirring occasionally, until the chard begins to wilt, about 2 minutes. Add the remaining chard, the juice of the lemon, and ¼ teaspoon salt. Cook until the chard is wilted, 2 to 3 minutes.

Divide the chard among the serving plates.

NUTRITIONAL STATS PER SERVING: 308 Calories, 47g Protein, 6g Carbohydrates, 11.5g Fat (1.5g Saturated), 112mg Cholesterol, 1g Sugar, 2g Fiber, 880mg Sodium

TOP NUTRIENTS: Vitamin C = 48%, Vitamin A = 43%, Magnesium = 26%, Potassium = 19%, Iron = 17%

REVIEW

Consider the following questions before you move on to Week 2:

1. Did you meet your goal for the week of adding 1 to 2 cups of greens each day?
2. Celebrate your successes! What approaches worked in helping you achieve that goal? What strategies could help as you move into next week?
3. Did you try any recipes? What skill could you work on to make cooking greens-based dishes easier for you?
4. How can you best continue to add greens to your meals as you move forward?

WEEK 2: RAINBOWS

When I ask patients to describe their typical plate, too often they paint me a mental picture full of boring beiges. Mother Nature created a world full of brightly colored fruits and vegetables—all with their own unique phytonutrients to promote health. These rainbows—sometimes referred to as "brainbows"—are chock-full of fiber and phytonutrients. Purple fruits and veggies, like eggplant and blueberries, boast phytonutrients called anthocyanins, which have amazing anti-inflammatory properties. Orange options, like carrots and sweet potatoes, get their sunny color from carotenoids, which convert into brain-boosting vitamin A. Reds—from strawberries to tomatoes—denote lycopene, an antioxidant dynamo of a nutrient. With so many incredible colors and tastes to choose from, why settle for beige?

Like greens, rainbow fruits and veggies should make up the bulk of your meals. Your goal is to add **1/2 cup or more of rainbows** to each meal.

How to Start

When reviewing your food assessment from Chapter 7 which rainbow fruits and veggies were regular players in your current diet? Where could you add more?

Vegetables can be challenging for some eaters. They don't like the taste or texture of vegetables and tend to gravitate toward basic options like carrots and broccoli. That's why one of the best ways to improve your rainbow consumption is to do an exercise we call "Build the Rainbow."

Consider the colors of the rainbow: purple, blue, green, yellow, orange, and red. First, list the fruits and vegetables in each color that you enjoy. Now, think about how you can build a rainbow into your veggie or fruit salad. Can you find a way to incorporate all six colors? What about in another dish like the Brainbow Kimchi Fried Rice (page 198)? The ultimate goal is to find ways to build a rainbow—or at least include fruits and/or vegetables of multiple colors—in each and every dish.

Tips and Tricks

One way to make sure you're getting enough of the rainbow is to shop with intention. Next time you're out shopping, take a good look around the produce section. There are so many exciting, colorful options; don't limit yourself! Why not branch out and try some purple sweet potatoes in the Crispy Pan-Seared Sweet Potatoes (page 196)? Maybe try a watermelon radish or radicchio? Grab a fresh avocado for some Crunchy Seedy Avocado Toast? There are so many delicious choices.

I'd also recommend having some frozen veggies—staples like onions, peas, peppers, and broccoli—on hand at all times. That makes it super easy to just grab a handful from the freezer when it's time to make a meal.

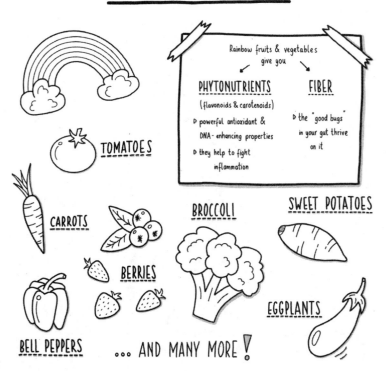

RAINBOWS

Rainbow fruits & vegetables give you

PHYTONUTRIENTS
(flavonoids & carotenoids)
▷ powerful antioxidant & DNA-enhancing properties
▷ they help to fight inflammation

FIBER
▷ the "good bugs" in your gut thrive on it

TOMATOES

CARROTS

BERRIES

BROCCOLI

SWEET POTATOES

EGGPLANTS

BELL PEPPERS ... AND MANY MORE!

Challenge

The biggest challenge most people face when it comes to increasing rainbow intake is simply knowing how to make these foods taste delicious. Too many of us were raised on mushy canned or boiled veggies. But you don't have to eat boiled peas for the rest of your life. Learning to cook vegetables in ways that minimize their nutrient loss and increase their flavor profile is a skill that can help you in your quest to eat to beat depression and anxiety. Try a fun sauté or stir-fry with as many rainbow colors as you can find. Savor meals punctuated by roasted brussels sprouts or cauliflower. And don't forget to rely on delicious sauces or dips to make rainbows more of a treat than a chore.

Crunchy Seedy Avocado Toast

SERVES 2

Toast, like pasta, is a food many people with anxiety and depression crave. To turn guilt-ridden carbs into brain-healthy toast, add a rainbow of phytonutrients and the many other benefits of the avocado, a wonderful source of monounsaturated fat. For a quick breakfast, add a poached egg or smoked salmon (or both!). Make a jar of toasted seeds to keep on hand and sprinkle them over the top or grab some everything bagel seasoning at the grocery store.

2 large slices sourdough bread

2 tablespoons olive-oil-based mayonnaise or softened unsalted butter

1 teaspoon poppy seeds

1 teaspoon sesame seeds

2 teaspoons pumpkin seeds (pepitas)

1 Haas avocado, thinly sliced

1/2 serrano chile, thinly sliced (or a pinch of red pepper flakes)

1 large radish, thinly sliced

2 tablespoons sprouts, microgreens, or finely chopped fresh herbs

1/2 large lemon

2 teaspoons sunflower seeds

Sea salt

Spread both sides of the bread with the mayonnaise. Sprinkle each side of the bread with the poppy, sesame, and pumpkin seeds, pressing them into the mayonnaise with your fingers or a spoon.

Warm a large skillet over medium heat. Place the seed-covered bread slices into the skillet and toast for 3 to 5 minutes, until golden brown. Flip and toast until golden brown on the second side.

Divide the avocado slices, chile slices, radish slices, and sprouts between the two slices of bread. Squeeze the lemon over both toasts. Garnish with the sunflower seeds and sprinkle with sea salt.

NUTRITIONAL STATS PER SERVING: 408 Calories, 9g Protein, 34g Carbohydrates, 28g Fat (3.5g Saturated), 6mg Cholesterol, 3g Sugars, 8g Fiber, 416mg Sodium

TOP NUTRIENTS: Thiamine = 41%, Folate = 39%, Vitamin B6 = 24%, Zinc = 24%, Selenium = 23%

Crispy Pan-Seared Sweet Potatoes

SERVES 6

Carb craving is often a part of depression, and finding ways to satisfy these cravings while giving your brain the nutrients it needs is part of the trick to eating to beat depression and anxiety. Rainbow plants tend to have healthier "slow carbs" along with their signature phytonutrients that fight inflammation. Crispy potatoes and seeds, creaminess from the tahini and feta, and a blast of herbaceousness combine to make this buffet of rainbows delicious. Purple sweet potatoes are one of my favorites and make this a striking dish—give them a try next time you see them at the market!

3 pounds sweet potatoes (4 medium, ideally no more than 2 to 2½ inches wide)

½ cup olive oil, divided, plus more as needed

Kosher salt

½ cup tahini

2 tablespoons fresh lemon juice

2 tablespoons warm water, plus more as needed

1 garlic clove, grated

¼ cup chopped soft herbs, such as cilantro, parsley, and basil

3 tablespoons seeds, such as sesame, pepita (pumpkin seeds), and sunflower

⅛ teaspoon red pepper flakes

Optional: 3 to 4 ounces feta cheese, crumbled

Preheat the oven to 425°F.

Place the sweet potatoes on a rimmed baking sheet and poke all over with a fork. Rub with ¼ cup of the olive oil. Sprinkle the skins with salt.

Roast for 45 minutes to 1 hour, until a paring knife slips in and out of a sweet potato easily. Be sure to check every sweet potato if they're different sizes.

Meanwhile, in a medium bowl, whisk the tahini, lemon juice, warm water, ½ teaspoon salt, and garlic until smooth. It will be very thick at first, but keep stirring! Add 1 tablespoon more warm water at a time as needed until you achieve a drizzle-able consistency.

Allow the sweet potatoes to cool for at least 20 minutes. Cut each sweet potato in half vertically, then use a fork to smash it, making craggy grooves in the flesh. It's okay if the skin rips a bit.

Warm the remaining ¼ cup of oil in a 12-inch (preferably cast-iron) skillet over medium heat. Working in batches so as not to overcrowd, add the sweet potatoes, flesh-side down, to the skillet. Resist the urge to smash them into the skillet—you want all of those craggy surfaces created with the fork to crisp up.

Cook for 3 to 4 minutes, until crispy and golden brown. Gently flip by sliding a spatula all the way under each potato and cook for 1 to 2 minutes on the skin side.

Transfer to a serving platter and repeat until all the sweet potatoes have been pan-fried. You will need to add more oil to the skillet between each round.

Drizzle the tahini sauce over the sweet potatoes, then top with herbs, seeds, and red pepper flakes. Finish with the cheese.

NUTRITIONAL STATS PER SERVING: 550 Calories, 12g Protein, 53g Carbohydrates, 34.5g Fat (7g Saturated), 15mg Cholesterol, 16g Sugars, 9g Fiber, 241mg Sodium

TOP NUTRIENTS: Vitamin A = 315%, Vitamin C = 64%, Vitamin B6 = 58%, Thiamine = 54%, Potassium = 26%

Roasted Shiitake and Spinach Grain Salad

SERVES 4

Grain salads and other healthy "slow carb" meals are a great vehicle for eating a lot of plants. Adding more fresh herbs to your meals is an easy way to improve nutrient density and make your cooking shine. Shiitake mushrooms add in more fiber and phytonutrients. This recipe uses the pasta-cooking method to cook the grains. Instead of perfect proportions of water to grains, just bring a huge pot of water to a boil as you would with pasta, then strain when done. By using this method you can cook any grains together—just time correctly!

This dish is great for making ahead, as it keeps for up to 5 days in the refrigerator.

1 pound shiitake mushrooms, stems removed and sliced ¼-inch thick

2 garlic cloves, minced

5 tablespoons extra-virgin olive oil, divided

Kosher salt and freshly ground black pepper

1 cup semi-pearled farro, rinsed

½ cup quinoa, rinsed

Juice of 1 large lemon (about 3 tablespoons)

1 tablespoon balsamic vinegar

2 cups fresh spinach leaves, roughly chopped

1 cup roughly chopped fresh basil leaves

3 ounces toasted pepitas (pumpkin seeds)

Optional: shaved Parmesan cheese

Preheat the oven to 325°F and line a rimmed baking sheet with parchment paper.

Toss the mushrooms and garlic with 2 tablespoons of olive oil, ¹/₂ teaspoon salt, and about ¹/₈ teaspoon pepper on the baking sheet. Spread the mushrooms into an even layer and roast until they are tender, about 30 minutes, stirring after 20 minutes.

Meanwhile, cook the farro and quinoa. Bring a large pot of salted water to a boil over high heat. Add the farro and cook for 5 minutes. Add the quinoa and cook for an additional 10 to 12 minutes, until the farro and quinoa are tender.

Drain and shake off as much water as possible. To cool the mixture quickly, spread evenly onto a baking sheet and place in the refrigerator. Otherwise, just leave it in the colander to cool.

Meanwhile, whisk 3 tablespoons olive oil, lemon juice, and vinegar together. Season with a small pinch of salt and pepper.

Toss the mushrooms, grains, lemon vinaigrette, spinach, and basil together in a large bowl. Season with salt and pepper.

Toss half of the pepitas into the salad and garnish with the remaining half and some cheese, if using.

NUTRITIONAL STATS PER SERVING: 490 Calories, 17g Protein, 48g Carbohydrates, 29g Fat (4.3g Saturated), 0mg Cholesterol, 4g Sugars, 8g Fiber, 100mg Sodium

TOP NUTRIENTS: Vitamin B6 = 33%, Zinc = 25%, Iron = 23%, Magnesium = 18%, Folate 16%

Brainbow Kimchi Fried Rice with Peanut Sauce

SERVES 4

Upgrade your plate with rainbows. That's a basic lesson in Nutritional Psychiatry, and this dish transforms fried rice from guilty takeout to all-star brain food. This is a great dish for eaters who find vegetables boring. Along with an array of colorful vegetables and bok choy, you get kimchi, a traditional fermented cabbage that adds probiotic power. You can use a wide variety of vegetables and greens to make this dish your own: sub in carrots, celery, fennel, asparagus, or any other dense vegetable for the bell pepper and bok choy, and spinach and chard in place of the bok choy. This recipe works with a variety of whole grains like barley and farro instead of rice. Anyone need a spicy peanut sauce to drizzle on top?

⅓ cup low-sodium soy sauce

¼ cup rice wine vinegar

2 tablespoons sriracha

2 tablespoons unsweetened, creamy peanut butter

3 tablespoons water, divided

2 teaspoons honey

2 tablespoons olive oil

1 large red bell pepper, finely chopped (about 1¼ cups)

1 large carrot, finely chopped (about 1 cup)

8 ounces bok choy, leaves roughly chopped, stems finely chopped

1 medium yellow onion, finely chopped

3 garlic cloves, minced

1 (1-inch) piece fresh ginger, grated or minced

3 cups cooked brown rice or other grain (preferably day-old)

2 large eggs

½ cup kimchi, chopped

Optional for garnish:
sriracha, sesame seeds, cilantro, chives, lime wedges

Whisk together the soy sauce, vinegar, sriracha, peanut butter, 2 tablespoons of water, and honey in a small bowl. Set aside.

Warm the olive oil in a 12-inch skillet over medium-high heat. Add the bell pepper, carrot, bok choy *stems only*, onion, and 1 tablespoon water and cook, stirring frequently with a wooden spoon, for 4 to 5 minutes, until almost tender. Stir in the garlic and ginger and cook for another 30 seconds.

Add the rice, bok choy greens, and peanut sauce and stir until everything is coated in the sauce and the greens are wilted.

Push the rice to the side to create a clearing in the skillet. Crack the eggs into the skillet and use the wooden spoon to scramble them rapidly. When the eggs are cooked, stir them into the rice.

Add the kimchi last to best preserve the live probiotic bacteria. Serve immediately.

NUTRITIONAL STATS PER SERVING: 421 Calories, 13g Protein, 60g Carbohydrates, 15.5g Fat (3g Saturated), 108mg Cholesterol, 12g Sugars, 7g Fiber, 1145mg Sodium

TOP NUTRIENTS: Vitamin C = 107%, Vitamin B6 = 56%, Vitamin A = 73%, Vitamin B1 = 37%, Magnesium = 37%

Turkey Zucchini Skillet Lasagna

SERVES 8

Lasagna is another one of our favorite comfort foods. In this case, we are bumping up the nutrient density by swapping out the noodles for zucchini. Salting the zucchini prevents the lasagna from being a bit watery. But you could skip this step and serve with a slotted spoon.

2 pounds zucchini

Kosher salt

1 tablespoon olive oil

1 small yellow onion, diced (about 1 cup)

1 pound ground dark turkey meat

4 garlic cloves, minced

2 (28-ounce) cans diced tomatoes

1 teaspoon dried oregano

1 teaspoon dried thyme

Freshly ground black pepper

2 cups fresh spinach, packed

16 ounces cottage cheese, drained

4 ounces mozzarella cheese, shredded (about 1 cup), divided

4 ounces Parmesan cheese, grated (about 1 cup), divided

1 egg

1/3 cup finely chopped fresh basil leaves, plus more for garnish

Cut the zucchini in half horizontally, then cut vertically into skinny strips. Spread the zucchini noodles out on several clean dish towels or paper towels and sprinkle both sides with salt. Let them sit until it's time to use the noodles, then pat totally dry.

Preheat the oven to 375°F.

Warm the olive oil in a 12-inch ovenproof skillet over medium-high heat. Add the onion and cook for 3 to 4 minutes, until slightly translucent. Add the ground turkey and garlic and cook, using a spoon to break the meat up into small pieces, until it is no longer pink, 4 to 5 minutes.

Stir in the diced tomatoes, oregano, and thyme. Season with 1/2 teaspoon salt and 1/4 teaspoon pepper. Lower the heat to medium and simmer for 10 to 15 minutes, stirring frequently, until the sauce has thickened significantly and no watery liquid remains on top. Stir in the spinach in batches.

Meanwhile, in a large bowl, combine the cottage cheese, 2 ounces (1/2 cup) of the mozzarella cheese, 2 ounces (1/2 cup) of the Parmesan cheese, the egg, basil, and 1/8 teaspoon pepper.

To assemble the lasagna, scoop all but a very thin layer of sauce out of the skillet and into a bowl. Layer the zucchini noodles over the top, overlapping as needed to cover the bottom of the skillet completely.

Top with one-third of the cottage cheese mixture and one-quarter of the remaining tomato mixture. Layer the zucchini noodles over the top, overlapping as necessary, and follow the same pattern two more times.

Cover the top layer of zucchini noodles completely with the remaining tomato sauce.

Bake uncovered for 40 minutes, then switch to broil. Sprinkle the remaining 2 ounces (½ cup) mozzarella cheese and 2 ounces (½ cup) Parmesan cheese over the top, place the skillet under the broiler, and broil for an additional 3 to 4 minutes to lightly brown the cheese.

Garnish with basil and pepper.

NUTRITIONAL STATS PER SERVING: 379 Calories, 28g Protein, 21g Carbohydrates, 20g Fat (8g Saturated), 96mg Cholesterol, 10g Sugars, 5g Fiber, 781mg Sodium

TOP NUTRIENTS: Vitamin C = 67%, Vitamin B6 = 23%, Potassium = 21%, Selenium 20%, Vitamin B12 = 18%

REVIEW

Consider the following questions before you move on to Week 3:

1. Did you meet your goal for the week of adding ½ cup rainbows to each meal?
2. Celebrate your successes! What approaches worked in helping you achieve that goal? What strategies could help you as you move into next week?
3. Did you try any recipes? What skill could you work on to make cooking rainbow-based dishes easier for you?
4. How can you best continue to add rainbow fruits and vegetables to your meals as you continue with the plan?

WEEK 3: SEAFOOD

There's no doubt that seafood is a challenging category for many people. It certainly was for me! However, it's one of the only ways to get those amazing omega-3 fatty acids like eicosapentaenoic acid (EPA) and docosahexaenoic acid (DHA), so this is a food category you should find a way to embrace. Those vital long-chain polyunsaturated fats (PUFAs) are amazing brain boosters and help stimulate the production of important nerve growth factors like brain-derived neurotrophic factor (BDNF), while also dampening inflammation across the body and brain. Seafood is also chock-full of other brain-healthy nutrients like iron, vitamin B12, zinc, and selenium. If you want to talk about eating for nutrient density, you really need look no further than a fresh piece of fish or bowl of mussels.

As someone who hadn't ventured beyond frozen fish sticks as a kid, I understand why adding **2 to 5 servings of seafood per week** can be a bit daunting. But once you find a way to include these delicious *fruits de mer* into your meal planning each week, you'll soon wonder why you worried. There's a lot of flavor and comfort to be found in a bowl of mussels diablo over pasta or a simple potato pancake with some smoked salmon and a little crème fraîche.

How to Start

As you look over your food assessment, where do you fall on the seafood spectrum? Are you someone who's already comfortable eating seafood? What about cooking it? Maybe you start by ordering the seafood special at your favorite restaurant or adding some fresh shrimp to your favorite brainbow salad. The simplest way to begin is to simply swap out chicken or beef for some type of seafood a couple of times each week.

Tips and Tricks

Your best bet with seafood is to buy fresh and cook it the same or next day. Frozen fish is also a great option, and more economical that fresh-caught, but it may taste or smell a bit fishier than fresher cuts. Thaw frozen fish overnight in the fridge. If you have a local fishmonger nearby, ask for recommendations about wild-caught, fresh fish options that are to your taste.

Remember, there are all types of ways to enjoy seafood. You don't have to cook up a big slab of white fish the way your grandma used to. You can try a nice fish taco or some noodles in dashi, a flavorful fish stock used in traditional Japanese cooking. Once you start experimenting, I think you'll see that adding this phenomenal brain food to your weekly menu planning is much easier than you thought.

Challenge

Many people remain concerned about mercury and microplastics—and for good reason. But these contaminants are much less of a risk when you opt for smaller fishes like sardines and anchovies. Mussels, clams, and oysters are great options to enjoy seafood without worry. There are hundreds of delicious ways to prepare seafood—from traditional ceviches to simple grilled fish steaks. Spend some time figuring out which methods work best for you.

Potato Pancakes with Smoked Salmon and Crème Fraîche

SERVES 4

Lox and other smoked, salted fish are traditional dishes that today are usually paired with bagels. Smoked salmon is an easy way to get more long-chain omega-3 fats into your meal plan. Look for lox made with wild salmon and without dyes. Oft maligned, potatoes are a good source of potassium and folate and create a nice base to balance the fish. These are wonderful for breakfast or as an appetizer.

2 tablespoons ground flax meal	2 teaspoons fresh thyme leaves
5 tablespoons water	½ teaspoon kosher salt
1½ pounds Yukon Gold potatoes	¼ teaspoon freshly ground black pepper
2 tablespoons all-purpose flour	8 teaspoons olive oil, divided
2 tablespoons minced fresh chives, plus more for garnish	8 ounces smoked salmon (about 8 slices)
	4 tablespoons crème fraîche

In a large bowl, mix together the flax meal and water. Allow to sit for at least 5 minutes to thicken up.

Grate the potatoes on the largest holes of a box grater into the center of a thin dish towel. Squeeze the towel as tight as you can over the sink to get out as much water as possible.

Add the potatoes, flour, chives, thyme, salt, and pepper to the bowl of flax and stir to combine.

Warm 2 teaspoons olive oil in a 10-inch skillet over medium heat. Working in batches, using one-quarter of the batter, make 4 potato pancakes by placing 4 equal dollops in the skillet and pressing down until each is about 8 inches wide. Cook for 5 to 6 minutes per side, until golden brown. Repeat, using more oil for each batch, until all the pancakes are cooked.

Divide the pancakes among 4 plates and top each with 2 ounces smoked salmon and 1 tablespoon crème fraîche. Garnish with chives.

NUTRITIONAL STATS PER SERVING: 328 Calories, 10g Protein, 35g Carbohydrates, 17g Fat (5g Saturated), 27mg Cholesterol, 2g Sugars, 5g Fiber, 407mg Sodium

TOP NUTRIENTS: Vitamin B6 = 77%, Vitamin C = 53%, Vitamin B12 = 42%, Potassium and Omega-3s (DHA+EPA) = 30%

Wild Salmon Burgers

Power-player salmon makes a serious burger, as it's a top source of long-chain omega-3 fats, B12, and protein for our mind and moods. Using canned wild salmon also takes away the pressure of buying the perfect fish or concerns about freshness, and it's a great value. A nice alternative to a typical beef burger, using salmon in this form is a perfect swap for eating to beat depression and anxiety. Adding phytonutrients to the burgers themselves with the dill, cilantro, green onion, ginger, and garlic boosts their brain-nutrient density even more. These burgers last a couple of days in the fridge once cooked, making them great for meal planning.

Dilly Wild Salmon Burgers

MAKES 4 BURGERS

2 large eggs

3 (5-ounce) cans wild salmon, drained

$\frac{1}{2}$ cup finely ground almond meal

1 organic lemon, zested and juiced

$\frac{1}{4}$ cup plus 2 tablespoons
  finely chopped fresh dill

2 tablespoons finely chopped fresh chives

Kosher salt and freshly ground black pepper

$\frac{1}{4}$ teaspoon garlic powder

$\frac{1}{3}$ cup plain whole-fat Greek yogurt

2 tablespoons extra-virgin olive oil, divided

For serving: 4 burger buns,
  sliced tomato, lettuce leaves,
  thinly sliced red onion

Whisk the eggs in a large bowl. Add the salmon and use a fork to smash it until no large chunks remain.

Add the almond meal, lemon zest, $\frac{1}{4}$ cup of the dill, the chives, $\frac{1}{2}$ teaspoon salt, $\frac{1}{8}$ teaspoon pepper, and the garlic powder and mix to combine. Form four $\frac{1}{2}$-inch-thick patties. Refrigerate if not cooking right away.

In a separate bowl, combine the yogurt, lemon juice, remaining 2 tablespoons dill, 1 tablespoon of the olive oil, $\frac{1}{4}$ teaspoon salt, and a pinch of pepper.

Warm the remaining 1 tablespoon of oil in a 12-inch skillet over medium-high heat. Cook the patties until golden brown all over, about 4 minutes per side.

Spread the dill sauce on the bottom of the burger buns, top with a salmon burger, more dill sauce, tomato, lettuce, and onion. Place the top bun on top and serve.

NUTRITIONAL STATS PER SERVING: 354 Calories, 30g Protein, 5g Carbohydrates, 24g Fat (4.5g Saturated), 180mg Cholesterol, 1g Sugar, 2g Fiber, 446mg Sodium

TOP NUTRIENTS: Selenium = 367%, Omega-3s (DHA+EPA) = 340% (1707mg), Vitamin B12 = 122%, Vitamin B6 = 112%, Vitamin A = 59%

Honey Soy Wild Salmon Burgers

MAKES 4 BURGERS

Yum! That's the general review of this burger. This fish burger is also dynamite covered with a cabbage slaw and wasabi mayo or sitting on top of a vegetable and brown rice bowl.

2 large eggs

3 (5-ounce) cans wild salmon, drained

½ cup panko breadcrumbs

2 tablespoons finely chopped fresh cilantro

2 green onions, minced

1 (1-inch) piece fresh ginger, peeled and grated

3 garlic cloves, grated

Juice of 1 large lime (about 3 tablespoons)

2 tablespoons low-sodium soy sauce

1 tablespoon extra-virgin olive oil

For serving: 4 burger buns, mayonnaise, 1 large thinly sliced avocado, lettuce leaves

Whisk the eggs in a large bowl. Add the salmon and use a fork to crush it up until no large chunks remain.

Add the panko, cilantro, green onions, ginger, garlic, lime juice, and soy sauce and mix to combine. Form four ½-inch-thick patties. Refrigerate if not cooking right away.

Warm the olive oil in a 12-inch skillet over medium-high heat. Cook the patties until golden brown all over, about 4 minutes per side.

Spread mayonnaise all over the cut sides of the burger buns. Add a salmon patty to each bun, then top with avocado and lettuce. Place the top bun on top and serve.

NUTRITIONAL STATS PER SERVING: 235 Calories, 28g Protein, 10g Carbohydrates, 8g Fat (1.5g Saturated), 174mg Cholesterol, 1g Sugar, 1g Fiber, 298mg Sodium

TOP NUTRIENTS: Selenium = 367%, Omega-3s (DHA+EPA) = 340% (1707mg), Vitamin B12 = 122%, Vitamin B6 =112%, Vitamin A = 59%

Mango-Ginger Shrimp Ceviche

SERVES 4

Worried about cooking seafood just right? This dish is your prescription. Ceviche is a traditional South American dish that uses the acid from lime juice to "cook" the fish, and versions exist on coasts around the world. If cooking a fillet of fish is intimidating or if you have tried ceviche but never made it at home, add this recipe to your lineup this week. The cooking instructions are for raw shrimp, but we make this in a jiffy using precooked wild shrimp, too. The kids love it and we can put a seafood meal on the table in minutes.

¾ cup fresh lime juice

¼ cup grapefruit juice

1 pound peeled, deveined raw wild shrimp

1 (1-inch) piece ginger, peeled and grated

1 large mango, diced

1 small red bell pepper, diced

½ jalapeño, sliced into very thin rounds

½ small red onion, finely minced

½ cup finely chopped fresh cilantro

Kosher salt

1 large avocado, diced

1 tablespoon extra-virgin olive oil

For serving: butter lettuce leaves, tortilla chips

Combine the lime juice and grapefruit juice and then divide it between two large bowls.

Chop the shrimp into ¼-inch pieces, add to one of the bowls, toss to coat, and place in the refrigerator for 20 minutes, but no longer. It will get tough if you "cook" it for too long.

To the other bowl, add the ginger, mango, bell pepper, jalapeño, red onion, cilantro, and ½ teaspoon salt and toss to combine.

Once the shrimp has been marinating for 20 minutes, pour the shrimp and juice into the other prepared bowl. Toss to combine. Taste and season with salt.

Top the ceviche with the diced avocado and olive oil. Season the avocado with a pinch of salt. Serve with butter lettuce leaves and/or tortilla chips.

NUTRITIONAL INFO PER SERVING: 244 Calories, 17g Protein, 24g Carbohydrates, 10.5g Fat (1.5g Saturated), 143mg Cholesterol, 14g Sugars, 5g Fiber, 348mg Sodium

TOP NUTRIENTS: Vitamin C = 108%, Vitamin B12 = 63%, Selenium = 62%, Vitamin B6 = 38%, Omega-3s (DHA+EPA) = 34%

Fish Tacos with Avocado Crema

SERVES 4

Seafood, rainbows, and leafy greens are often eaten with a side of beans. Fish tacos are the complete package and a game changer for your seafood consumption. After all, it's your taco, so toppings are totally up to you. This recipe upgrades the standard cabbage and fried fish combo with a lovely avocado crema and pairs it with arugula, corn, cilantro, and tomato for a summery rainbow taco dream. Other quick toppings: sliced peppers, pico de gallo, pickled jalapeño, and radish.

Fish Tacos

- 1 cup club soda
- 1/2 cup cassava flour
- 2 tablespoons tapioca flour or cornstarch
- 1 1/2 teaspoons kosher salt
- 1 teaspoon smoked paprika
- 1 teaspoon onion powder
- 1/2 teaspoon garlic powder
- 1/4 cup neutral cooking oil, such as avocado, grapeseed, or refined coconut
- 1 1/2 pounds skinned cod, cut into 3-inch pieces
- 8 corn tortillas
- 1 1/2 cups baby arugula
- 2 ears of cooked corn, kernels removed
- 1 large Roma tomato, diced
- 1/2 small white onion, diced
- 1/2 cup chopped fresh cilantro

Avocado Crema

- 1 large Haas avocado
- 1/3 cup plain Greek yogurt or sour cream
- Juice of 1 large lime (about 2 tablespoons)
- 1/4 teaspoon kosher salt
- 1/8 teaspoon garlic powder

To make the fish tacos:

In a large bowl, whisk the club soda, cassava flour, tapioca flour, salt, paprika, onion powder, and garlic powder until smooth. It will be a very loose, thin batter, just thicker than heavy cream.

Warm the neutral oil in a large skillet over medium-high heat. When you flick a drop of water into it and it sizzles immediately, it's ready. Add about one-third of the fish to the batter and stir gently with a fork to coat.

Pick up each piece with a fork, allowing excess batter to drip off, and add to the skillet. Don't overcrowd the skillet. Cook for 2 to 3 minutes per side, until golden brown. Transfer to a paper towel–lined plate, sprinkle with salt, and continue cooking the rest of the fish.

To make the avocado crema:

Combine the avocado, yogurt, lime juice, salt, and garlic powder in a bowl and mash and whisk until smooth. It's okay if it's a little lumpy.

To serve:

To warm the tortillas, either char them by placing them directly over the open flame of a gas stove over medium-low heat for about 20 seconds per side or wrap the entire stack in damp paper towels and microwave for 25 seconds.

Place the arugula in the center of each tortilla, then top with fried fish, avocado crema, corn, tomato, onion, and cilantro. Enjoy immediately.

NUTRITIONAL STATS PER SERVING: 575 Calories, 36g Protein, 53g Carbohydrates, 25.5g Fat (5g Saturated), 83mg Cholesterol, 5g Sugars, 8g Fiber, 974mg Sodium

TOP NUTRIENTS: Selenium = 105%, Vitamin B6 = 77%, Omega-3s (DHA+EPA) = 66%, Vitamin B12 = 63%, Potassium = 46%

Soba Dashi with Poached Egg

SERVES 4

Dashi is a traditional Japanese healing broth made of kombu seaweed and smoked, fermented, dried fish flakes called bonito. This simple broth can be adorned with an array of plants, fermented foods, and seafood, making it a great dish for your kitchen. We top with power-player eggs for a dose of choline and perfect protein. Top with fresh, raw, crunchy veggies or stir in a big handful of spinach, sliced bok choy, or zucchini noodles to cook at the last minute. It is very easy to poach the eggs right in the broth, but if you'd rather soft- or hard-boil your eggs, go that route.

8 cups water

2 (4-inch) squares kombu seaweed

3 tablespoons bonito flakes

3 tablespoons low-sodium soy sauce

2 tablespoons sesame oil

2 tablespoons rice wine vinegar

2 teaspoons sriracha or other hot sauce

8 ounces dried soba noodles

4 large eggs

1 cup shredded carrots

½ cup thinly sliced scallions

½ cup thinly sliced radishes

2 teaspoons sesame seeds

Combine the water, kombu, and bonito flakes in a large saucepan and bring to a boil over high heat. Remove from the heat and allow the kombu and bonito to steep for 20 to 30 minutes.

Strain the broth using a fine-mesh strainer placed over a large bowl. Rinse out the saucepan if needed, then return the broth to the pan.

Bring the broth to a boil over high heat, then stir in the soy sauce, sesame oil, vinegar, and sriracha and reduce the heat to medium-low.

Stir in the noodles and cook for 1 minute. Push the noodles to one side of the saucepan. Crack the eggs, one at a time, into a small bowl, then gently slip them into the water. Cover the pot and cook for 4 to 5 minutes, until the egg whites are set but the yellows are still runny.

Divide the eggs, noodles, and broth among 4 bowls. Top with the carrots, scallions, radishes, and sesame seeds.

NUTRITIONAL STATS PER SERVING: 371 Calories, 15g Protein, 52g Carbohydrates, 12g Fat (2g Saturated), 175mg Cholesterol, 6g Sugars, 2g Fiber, 423mg Sodium

TOP NUTRIENTS: Vitamin B12 = 63%, Thiamine = 45%, Vitamin A = 40%, Choline = 28%, Folate = 22%

Simple Steamed Clams with Fresh Herbs and Lemon

SERVES 4

Clams are a superfood and nature's most concentrated source of vitamin B12. An original human brain food, for years people have reported a kind of buzz after eating bivalves. Maybe it's the minerals, maybe it's the B vitamins, but it seems the brain recognizes clams. It's doctor recommended to serve with a good baguette for dipping in the sauce. For a crowd, create a mini clambake by adding 2 ears of corn that have been cut into 6 pieces and a pound of 1-inch sliced andouille sausage to the pot when you add the clams.

2 tablespoons extra virgin olive oil

1 large shallot, minced

4 garlic cloves, thinly sliced

5 pounds clams, preferably littleneck

2 tablespoons unsalted butter

Zest and juice of 1 large lemon (about 3 tablespoons)

2 tablespoons minced fresh basil

2 tablespoons minced fresh parsley

2 tablespoons minced fresh chives

¼ teaspoon red pepper flakes

Kosher salt

Warm the olive oil in a large Dutch oven or other wide pot over medium heat. Add the shallot and garlic and cook for 3 to 4 minutes, until softened.

Add the clams and cover the pot. Cook for 6 to 10 minutes, until most of the clams are open. Use a slotted spoon to transfer the open clams to a serving bowl. Discard any clams that are still closed.

With the heat still on medium, add the butter, lemon zest, lemon juice, basil, parsley, chives, and red pepper flakes to the skillet (which is now full of clam juice) and stir to combine for about 1 minute. Taste and season with salt.

Pour the sauce over the clams and serve immediately.

NUTRITIONAL STATS PER SERVING: 335 Calories, 37g Protein, 11g Carbohydrates, 15g Fat (4.5g Saturated), 90mg Cholesterol, 1g Sugar, 568mg Sodium

TOP NUTRIENTS: Vitamin B12 = 1750%, Vitamin A = 72%, Iron = 66%, Omega-3s (DHA+EPA) = 40% (200mg), Selenium = 38%

REVIEW

Consider the following questions before you move on to Week 4:

1. Did you meet your goal for the week of 2 to 3 seafood meals?
2. Celebrate your successes! What approaches worked in helping you achieve that goal? What strategies could help you as you move into next week?
3. Did you try any recipes? What skill could you work on to make cooking seafood dishes easier for you?
4. How can you best continue to add seafood to your meals as you move forward?

SEAFOOD

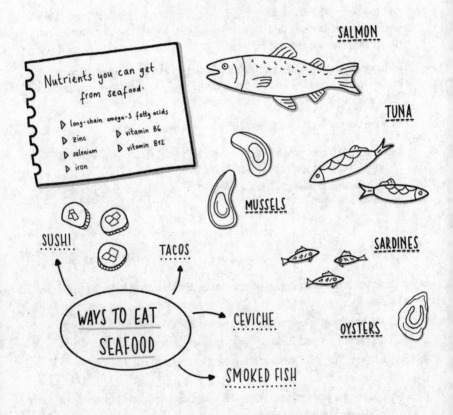

Nutrients you can get from seafood:
- long-chain omega-3 fatty acids
- zinc
- selenium
- iron
- vitamin B6
- vitamin B12

SALMON

TUNA

MUSSELS

SARDINES

OYSTERS

SUSHI

TACOS

CEVICHE

SMOKED FISH

WAYS TO EAT SEAFOOD

WEEK 4: NUTS, BEANS, AND SEEDS

This brain food category is generally underrepresented in the average person's diet. And that's too bad, as these foods are not only a great way to add some extra fiber to your diet but they also provide much-needed phytonutrients and plant-based proteins. The other great thing about this category? It's an easy add. Replace your go-to sugary or salty midafternoon snack with a handful of raw almonds to not only sate your hunger but also help boost your brain function. Throw a handful of beans or pepitas (pumpkin seeds) in your favorite salad or in a bowl of soup. Try a serving of walnuts or cashews in your smoothies for a little additional unexpected creaminess—as well as an extra shot of plant-based protein. There's really no end to how you can use this food category to increase nutrient density in your meals.

When you start to think about all the ways that nuts, seeds, and legumes are used in dishes, you'll probably realize you already have a few favorites to choose from. Who doesn't love a hot, nourishing cup of lentil soup on a winter's day? Or a delicious hummus dip paired with fresh veggies or whole-grain crackers? Like greens, nuts, beans, and seeds can easily add that little something extra to your favorite meals. Try to find ways to add **at least a small handful** of these foods to your meals or as a stand-alone snack each day.

How to Start

When referring back to your food assessment, you may notice that you are not eating much in the way of nuts, beans, and seeds. If so, you're not alone. But, as stated, these foods are very easy to swap in for popular snacks or to add to your favorite dishes. They're also helpful for sating your sweet tooth. Trying the Buckwheat Cacao Pancakes (page 215) or Chocolate Brain Truffles (page 220) are great ways to consume foods from this category with just the right touch of sweetness.

Tips and Tricks

Chances are, you already have a favorite soup or chili recipe that calls for beans. Instead of sticking with one type, try adding in different varieties; you can create a rainbow just in beans alone without much effort.

Nuts make a great snack. Having raw varieties on hand for that midafternoon pick-me-up or to help you coast between meals is easy. They're also great additions to salads, soups, and other dishes. Before you know it, you'll be tossing them into your favorites with abandon.

Challenge

Many people are concerned about the high fat and calorie content of nuts. Remember, a little goes a long way—and buying raw cashews, almonds, or walnuts is generally the best way to go to help keep your energy levels up throughout the day without too much fat or sodium.

Buckwheat Cacao Pancakes with Raspberry Compote

MAKES 12 PANCAKES

Pancakes are a comfort food, and this version is energizing and mood boosting. With ample fiber and magnesium, these pancakes are great for the microbiome and mental health. Using cacao nibs brings all the benefits of chocolate and none of the sugar. Instead, we've added banana for sweetness and potassium. Buckwheat flour is gluten-free and has ten times more magnesium than white flour. To make a vegan version, use your preferred milk substitute and a flax egg in place of the egg by whisking 1 tablespoon ground flax with 2½ tablespoons water and letting it sit for five minutes.

Compote

- ½ pound fresh or frozen raspberries
- 1 tablespoon lemon juice
- 1 tablespoon maple syrup
- ¼ teaspoon pure vanilla extract
- 2 teaspoons chia seeds

Pancakes

- 1 ripe banana
- 1 cup whole milk
- 1 tablespoon fresh lemon juice
- 1 tablespoon maple syrup, plus more for serving
- 1 tablespoon avocado or coconut oil, plus more for cooking
- 1 large egg, whisked
- 1 teaspoon pure vanilla extract
- 1 cup buckwheat flour
- 1 teaspoon baking powder
- ½ teaspoon kosher salt
- ½ cup cacao nibs
- **Optional:** grass-fed butter

First, get the compote started. Add the raspberries, lemon juice, maple syrup, and vanilla extract to a small saucepan and bring the mixture to a boil over medium-high heat. Stir often. Reduce to medium-low heat. Keep stirring and use a fork or whisk to mash the fruit. When it has reduced by about half and is quite thick, stir in the chia seeds and set aside to cool slightly.

In a medium bowl, use a fork to mash the banana thoroughly. Stir in the milk and lemon juice and allow to sit for at least 10 minutes to create your own buttermilk. (Alternatively, you can just use 1 cup of buttermilk and skip the lemon juice.)

Stir the maple syrup, avocado oil, egg, and vanilla into the milk mixture.

In a separate larger bowl, whisk together buckwheat flour, baking powder, and salt.

Stir the wet ingredients into the dry ingredients until just combined. Don't over-mix or the pancakes will be tough! Let the batter rest for at least 5 minutes.

Warm a large skillet over medium heat. Add 1 tablespoon avocado oil and swirl to coat the skillet. Use a ¼-cup scoop or measuring cup to add pancake batter to the skillet. Sprinkle each pancake with cacao nibs.

Flip when bubbles form on the pancakes and then pop, 3 to 4 minutes. Cook until the second side is golden brown, 1 to 2 minutes. Repeat until all the pancake batter is cooked.

Top with raspberry compote. Serve with maple syrup and butter if desired.

NUTRITIONAL STATS PER SERVING (3 PANCAKES): 350 Calories, 8g Protein, 41g Carbohydrates, 16.5g Fat (8g Saturated), 51mg Cholesterol, 10g Sugars, 11g Fiber, 286mg Sodium

TOP NUTRIENTS: Magnesium = 34%, Vitamin B12 = 21%, Choline = 8%, Vitamin A = 8%, Iron = 6%, Vitamin C = 6%

Coconut-Ginger Lentil Soup

SERVES 4

Lentils are a staple of eating to beat depression and anxiety, as they are an excel-lent source of folate, fiber, and plant-based protein. Combining top food catego-ries, like the spinach in this recipe, always ensures high nutrient density. Ginger and turmeric are closely related plants with an array of unique anti-inflammatory phytonutrients including turmeric's curcumin. Lentil soup is on our menu weekly, often a vegetarian version using vegetable broth or even just water.

1 tablespoon coconut oil

1 large red bell pepper, diced

1 medium yellow onion, diced

1 cup dried red lentils

4 garlic cloves, grated

1 (2-inch) piece ginger, peeled and grated

½ teaspoon ground turmeric

½ teaspoon paprika

¼ teaspoon red pepper flakes

3 cups chicken broth or bone broth

1 (14.5-ounce) can diced tomatoes

1 (13.5-ounce) can unsweetened coconut milk

Kosher salt

3 cups fresh spinach, chopped
(3½ to 4 ounces)

⅓ cup finely chopped fresh basil
leaves, plus more for garnish

Juice of 1 large lemon (about
3 tablespoons)

Optional: plain yogurt, for topping

Warm the coconut oil in a large heavy-bottomed pot over medium-high heat. Add the bell pepper and onion and cook until softened, 3 to 4 minutes. Add the lentils, garlic, ginger, turmeric, paprika, and red pepper flakes and cook for an additional 1 minute.

Stir in the broth, tomatoes, coconut milk, and 1 teaspoon salt. Bring to a boil over high heat, then reduce the heat to medium-low and cook for 20 to 25 minutes, until the lentils are tender.

Stir in the spinach and basil and cook until wilted. Taste and season with additional salt if needed. Stir in the lemon juice just before serving. Top with basil leaves and yogurt, if using.

NUTRITIONAL STATS PER SERVING: 303 Calories, 15g Protein, 47g Carbohydrates, 7g Fat (4.5g Saturated), 4mg Cholesterol, 7g Sugars, 10g Fiber, 931mg Sodium

TOP NUTRIENTS: Vitamin C = 111%, Folate = 46%, Vitamin B6 = 36%, Zinc = 31%, Thiamine = 31%, Iron = 28%

Mushroom and Chicken Cassoulet

SERVES 6

Great for batch cooking, one-pot meals are a simple solution for more brain food. This combination of beans, chicken, and mushrooms is extra satisfying and filling thanks to fiber from the beans and mushrooms. Mushrooms, like beans, are an underconsumed brain food and contain high amounts of fiber, potassium, and unique phytonutrients, many of which are being researched regarding their impact on brain health. The pepita-pecorino breadcrumbs give this an incredible umami crunch plus a dash of zinc and magnesium. (If you love this crunch, try it on the All Kale Caesar, page 180.) Instead of the chicken, double the mushrooms and beans for a vegetarian cassoulet. For an even richer version, make the sauce with a half pound of Italian sausage.

1 tablespoon olive oil

1 pound boneless, skinless chicken
 thighs, cut into 1-inch cubes

Kosher salt and freshly ground black pepper

1 shallot, diced

8 ounces oyster mushrooms,
 roughly chopped

2 large carrots, diced

6 garlic cloves, minced

1 (28-ounce) can diced tomatoes

1 (15-ounce) can great northern
 beans, drained and rinsed

4 thyme sprigs

1 bay leaf

1/2 teaspoon dried oregano

1/4 teaspoon red pepper flakes

1/2 cup finely chopped fresh parsley leaves

4 tablespoons unsalted butter

1 cup panko breadcrumbs

1/2 cup pepitas (pumpkin
 seeds), finely chopped

1/2 cup grated pecorino Romano cheese

Warm the olive oil in a 12-inch ovenproof skillet (preferably cast-iron) over medium-high heat.

Season the chicken with 1 teaspoon salt and 1/4 teaspoon pepper. Cook for 3 minutes per side to sear. Transfer to a holding plate. It's okay if it's not totally cooked through.

Add the shallot, mushrooms, and carrots and cook until the liquid has evaporated from the mushrooms, 7 to 9 minutes. Add the garlic and cook, stirring constantly, for another 30 seconds.

Stir in the tomatoes, beans, cooked chicken, thyme sprigs, bay leaf, oregano, red pepper flakes, and 1/2 teaspoon salt. Reduce the heat to medium-low and simmer, stirring often, for 10 minutes, or until the excess liquid has evaporated. Stir in the parsley, then remove the skillet from the heat and use a spatula to smooth the top.

Meanwhile, melt the butter in a small skillet over medium heat. Add the panko, pepitas, and 1/4 teaspoon salt and stir until combined. Stir in the cheese until it is melted and combined with the breadcrumbs.

Scatter the breadcrumbs over the cassoulet and transfer the skillet to the oven. Bake for 20 to 25 minutes, until the breadcrumbs are golden brown.

Allow to cool for several minutes, then pick out and discard the thyme sprigs and bay leaf and serve.

NUTRITIONAL STATS PER SERVING: 619 Calories, 48g Protein, 53g Carbohydrates, 25g Fat (11.5g Saturated), 110mg Cholesterol, 7g Sugars, 11g Fiber, 746mg Sodium

TOP NUTRIENTS: Vitamin A = 65%, Vitamin C = 39%, Folate = 32%, Thiamine = 25%, Vitamin B6 = 25%, Potassium = 22%

Red Bean Hummus

SERVES 4

Beans are easy on the budget and great for brain health from their combination of B vitamins, protein, magnesium, and microbiome-fueling fiber. Learn to use dried beans, either soaking and cooking on the stovetop or pressure cooking for incredible value, or use canned organic beans. This version uses red kidney beans, but you can use any kind of bean you want—black beans, cannellini, or the classic chickpeas. Soaking the garlic in the lemon juice while prepping lessens its bite. For extra kick, add cayenne.

¼ cup fresh lemon juice

1 garlic clove, peeled

2 cups cooked kidney beans

¼ cup tahini

1 teaspoon lemon zest

½ teaspoon kosher salt

¼ teaspoon ground cumin

1 tablespoon extra-virgin olive oil

1 tablespoon chopped pepitas
(pumpkin seeds)

Combine the lemon juice and garlic in a food processor and allow to sit for 10 minutes.

Add the kidney beans, tahini, lemon zest, salt, and cumin to the food processor and process until smooth, about 20 seconds. If needed, add 1 tablespoon of water at a time until the desired consistency is achieved.

Transfer to a serving bowl and drizzle with the olive oil. Sprinkle with the pepitas and serve with crunchy vegetables like celery and carrots or your favorite whole-grain, seedy cracker.

NUTRITIONAL STATS PER SERVING: 227 Calories, 9g Protein, 19g Carbohydrates, 14g Fat (2g Saturated), 0mg Cholesterol, 2g Sugars, 8g Fiber, 254mg Sodium

TOP NUTRIENTS: Folate = 34%, Magnesium = 26%, Zinc = 25%, Iron = 21%, Potassium = 11%

Chocolate Brain Truffles

MAKES 24 TRUFFLES

Examining your relationship with dark chocolate is important in moving beyond treats and cheats as an eater. Dark chocolate is a power player for brain health, as you learned on page 110, for its flavanols, fiber, and minerals. These truffles add the brain health benefits of nuts, seeds, and whole grains that makes for a winning combo. You can use any combination of nut butter or seeds you like—some of my favorites are almond butter and chopped pistachios or peanut butter and pecans. If you need more cacao in your brain, you can dip the truffles in melted chocolate or dust with cacao powder. For folks with nut allergies, swap in sunflower butter for the nut butter.

½ cup rolled oats	12 ounces (about 20) Medjool dates, pitted
½ cup unsweetened coconut flakes	¾ cup cashew butter
2 tablespoons hemp seeds	1 teaspoon vanilla extract
2 tablespoons chia seeds	¼ cup dark chocolate chunks
⅛ teaspoon kosher salt	½ cup cacao nibs

Combine the oats, coconut, hemp seeds, chia seeds, and salt in a food processor and process until finely ground. Add the dates, cashew butter, and vanilla and process until the mixture starts to clump up into a ball.

Add the chocolate chunks and cacao nibs and pulse 15 to 20 times to chop up the chocolate and incorporate it into the dough.

Roll the dough into tablespoon-sized balls.

Place the dough balls on a parchment-lined baking sheet and freeze until hard, about 1 hour. Transfer to a storage container and keep in the refrigerator.

Let the truffles sit at room temperature for a couple of minutes before enjoying.

NUTRITIONAL STATS PER SERVING (2 TRUFFLES): 284 Calories, 4g Protein, 34g Carbohydrates, 16g Fat (6g Saturated), 0mg Cholesterol, 22g Sugars, 6g Fiber, 70mg Sodium

TOP NUTRIENTS: Magnesium = 37%, Zinc = 19%, Iron = 16%, Potassium = 9%, Selenium = 6%

NUTS, BEANS & SEEDS

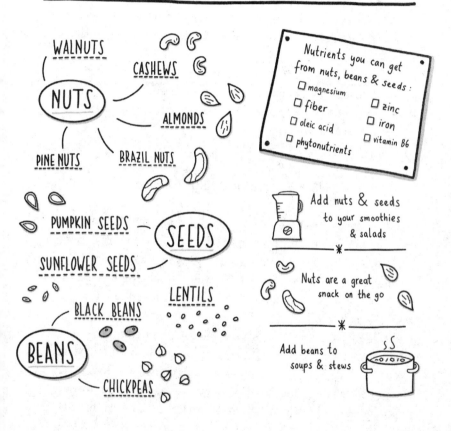

WALNUTS

CASHEWS

NUTS

ALMONDS

PINE NUTS

BRAZIL NUTS

PUMPKIN SEEDS

SEEDS

SUNFLOWER SEEDS

LENTILS

BLACK BEANS

BEANS

CHICKPEAS

Nutrients you can get from nuts, beans & seeds:

☐ magnesium
☐ fiber   ☐ zinc
☐ oleic acid   ☐ iron
☐ phytonutrients   ☐ vitamin B6

Add nuts & seeds to your smoothies & salads

Nuts are a great snack on the go

Add beans to soups & stews

WEEK 5: GOOD MICROBIOME BUGS

You've spent the last four weeks adding foods that help support your microbiome by providing it the fiber it needs to thrive. But to continually seed the gut with good bugs, you'll also benefit from adding some fermented foods to your diet. Including live-culture foods like kefir, yogurt, miso, kombucha, and sauerkraut is a great way to do just that.

While many of these foods are staples in other cultures, the traditional Western diet doesn't put a high premium on fermented foods. You may not be as familiar with ferments, and that's okay. Here's your chance to find delicious ways to add **three to five servings** of fermented foods each week in service of your microbiome—and your brain.

How to Start

Do you already enjoy fermented foods? Which ones? Are there places you could replace traditional dairy with natural, full-fat kefir or yogurt? The Chocolate Peanut Butter Cup Smoothie (page 225) is a tasty way to start. And who doesn't love a great grilled cheese sandwich with bacon? You can turn this food into a brain-boosting meal with the simple addition of some sauerkraut.

Tips and Tricks

Kefir and yogurt are easy additions to a morning smoothie, of course. But miso soup, like the butternut squash variety in the recipe on page 226, or seared pork chops with sauerkraut (page 227) are also satisfying ways to indulge in this food category.

Challenge

Familiarity is usually the biggest barrier to entry here. You want to make sure you don't accidentally stock up on fermented foods that are full of sugar and other additives and preservatives. And be sure to buy fermented foods with live cultures, which will be refrigerated in the grocery store, as opposed to "pickled" foods on the shelf which are simply preserved in vinegar.

Make sure to pick up plain, full-fat kefir and yogurt with no added sugar and then add your own sweetness with honey, berries, or a little dark chocolate to taste.

Healthy-Brain Smoothie

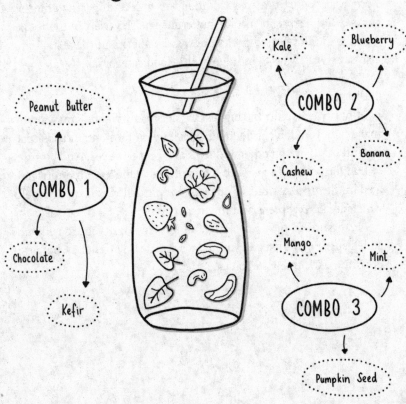

Chocolate Peanut Butter Cup Smoothie

MAKES 1 SMOOTHIE

Beating depression and anxiety with food means more beans and legumes . . . like cacao beans and peanut butter. Smoothies are great for brain nutrition when appetites and motivation are low. If the sourness of the kefir needs to be sweetened beyond the banana, add a date or a drizzle of honey. This recipe works well with yogurt, too—add a splash of liquid to achieve your desired consistency. If you forgot to freeze the banana, add a handful of ice.

¾ cup plain full-fat kefir

¼ cup water

1 cup packed fresh spinach

1 banana, cut into 1-inch pieces and frozen

2 tablespoons cacao powder

2 tablespoons peanut butter

2 Brazil nuts

¼ teaspoon almond extract

1 teaspoon cacao nibs, for garnish

In the following order, put the kefir, water, spinach, banana, cacao powder, peanut butter, Brazil nuts, and almond extract into a high-powered blender. Blend for 30 to 45 seconds, until all the ingredients are incorporated. Pour into a glass, top with the cacao nibs, and serve immediately.

NUTRITIONAL STATS PER SERVING: 515 Calories, 19g Protein, 56g Carbohydrates, 24.5g Fat (5g Saturated), 9mg Cholesterol, 30g Sugars, 9g Fiber, 229mg Sodium

TOP NUTRIENTS: Selenium = 283%, Magnesium = 64%, B6 = 54%, Potassium = 27%, Vitamin A = 65%, Vitamin B12 = 23%

Kefir Berry Smoothie

MAKES 1 SMOOTHIE

Berries have their brain food reputation for good reasons. These low glycemic fruits are loaded with phytonutrients linked to improved brain health. And while berries get the headline, nuts and seeds are the secret all-stars to a brain food smoothie, offering fiber and slow-burning carbs to balance out the sugars of the fruit. Kefir contains more CFUs (colony-forming units) of the good bugs that are central to microbiome health, quelling inflammation and improving mental fitness.

¾ cup plain full-fat kefir

⅓ cup white beans

⅓ cup water

1½ cups frozen blueberries

½ large banana

½ cup chopped spinach

2 tablespoons raw, unsalted almonds

2 tablespoons raw, unsalted pepitas (pumpkin seeds)

In the following order, put the kefir, beans, water, blueberries, banana, spinach, almonds, and pepitas into a high-powered blender. Blend for 30 to 45 seconds, until all the ingredients are incorporated. Pour into a glass and serve immediately.

NUTRITIONAL STATS PER SERVING: 461 Calories, 19g Protein, 64g Carbohydrates, 18g Fat (3g Saturated), 9mg Cholesterol, 36g Sugars, 14g Fiber, 96mg Sodium

TOP NUTRIENTS: Magnesium = 89%, Vitamin A = 70%, Folate = 45%, Potassium = 32%, Vitamin C = 25%

Miso Butternut Squash Soup

SERVES 4

Soups are an essential tool for eating to beat depression and anxiety. Nutrient rich, soothing, and calming, we boost this butternut soup with miso, a fermented soybean paste, adding in more protein, fiber, and good bugs. No immersion blender? Wait until the soup has cooled significantly, then add to a blender in batches and blend until smooth.

2 tablespoons coconut or olive oil

1 medium yellow onion, roughly chopped

4 garlic cloves, chopped

2½ pounds butternut squash, roughly chopped (1 medium butternut squash)

5 to 6 cups low-sodium vegetable broth

¼ cup raw cashews

2 tablespoons soy sauce

Kosher salt

¼ cup white miso paste

Juice of 1 large lime (about 2 tablespoons)

Warm the coconut oil in a large heavy-bottomed pot over medium heat. Add the onion and cook for 3 to 4 minutes, until softened. Add the garlic and cook for 1 more minute.

Stir in the squash, 5 cups of the broth, the cashews, soy sauce, and ½ teaspoon salt. Bring to a boil over high heat, then reduce the heat to medium-low, cover, and cook for 20 to 30 minutes, until the squash is very tender.

Remove the pot from the heat, stir in the miso and lime juice, and blend with an immersion blender until completely smooth. Add more broth if needed to achieve your desired consistency.

NUTRITIONAL STATS PER SERVING: 284 Calories, 6g Protein, 46g Carbohydrates, 10.5 Fat (6g Saturated), 0mg Cholesterol, 12g Sugars, 7g Fiber, 1064mg Sodium

TOP NUTRIENTS: Vitamin A = 215%, Vitamin C = 87%, Potassium = 23%, Thiamine = 27%, Vitamin B6 = 39%

One-Skillet Pork Chops with Plums and Red Onion

SERVES 4

Pork and sauerkraut are a classic pairing, and this one-skillet dish is a satisfying explosion of flavor, thiamine, zinc, and vitamin B12. The plums and red onions cook down into a delicious base. Add a side of brown rice or farro if you need to bulk it up on a hungry night. This recipe is a model—use what's in season or what you've got on hand. Yellow onion will do the trick in place of red, and you can swap any stone fruit for the plums. Just don't forget the sauerkraut, which balances the sweetness of the plum mixture and adds plenty of good bugs. Look for local, pasture-raised pork.

4 (1½-inch-thick) boneless pork chops

Kosher salt and freshly ground black pepper

2 tablespoons olive oil, divided

1 large red onion, sliced ¼-inch thick

4 large garlic cloves, thinly sliced

4 large plums, sliced ½-inch thick

1 tablespoon apple cider vinegar

1 tablespoon unsalted butter

2 teaspoons Dijon mustard, plus more for serving

½ cup sauerkraut

Season the pork chops generously (as in, way more than you think!) with salt and pepper and allow to rest at room temperature for 30 minutes.

Heat a 12-inch skillet, preferably cast-iron, over medium-high heat for several minutes. Add 1 tablespoon of olive oil and warm for 30 seconds. Turn on your over-the-stove vent, as the pork chops will get very smoky. Cook the pork chops for 3 minutes per side, or until an instant-read thermometer registers 135°F. If the sides look pink, use tongs to turn and sear each side for about 30 seconds. Transfer the pork chops to a holding plate and reduce the heat to medium.

When the skillet has cooled for a few minutes, add the remaining 1 tablespoon oil, the red onion, and garlic. Season with salt and pepper. Cook for about 5 minutes, stirring often, until the onions are soft but not totally shapeless. Add the plums and cook for 3 to 4 minutes, until they are soft and warm but not mushy. Remove the skillet from the heat and stir in the vinegar, butter, and mustard until incorporated.

Nestle the pork chops down into the warm plums to rewarm if needed.

Serve the pork chops over the plum and onion mixture, with a dollop of mustard and 2 tablespoons of sauerkraut alongside.

NUTRITIONAL STATS PER SERVING: 551 Calories, 56g Protein, 12g Carbohydrates, 31g Fat (8g Saturated), 178mg Cholesterol, 8g Sugars, 2g Fiber, 409mg Sodium

TOP NUTRIENTS: Selenium = 155%, Thiamine = 106%, Zinc = 94%, Vitamin B6 = 94%, Vitamin B12 = 60%

Kimchi Pancakes

MAKES 8 PANCAKES

Comforting for your mood and your microbiome, these savory pancakes are a great vehicle for eating more plants. Kimchi is a traditional Korean dish of fermented cabbage with many variations that you can find in the grocery store. These pancakes make eating fermented foods an easy habit to form.

Pancakes

1 large egg

1¼ cups all-purpose flour

⅓ cup water

1 tablespoon kimchi brine

2 tablespoons rice wine vinegar

1 tablespoon low-sodium soy sauce

1 cup kimchi, finely chopped

1 cup red bell pepper, sliced into
1½-inch long thin slices

1 teaspoon sesame seeds

½ teaspoon kosher salt

2 to 3 tablespoons avocado oil, divided

Dipping Sauce

2 tablespoons soy sauce or coconut aminos

2 tablespoons rice wine vinegar

1 teaspoon honey

¼ teaspoon sesame seeds

Whisk the egg in a large bowl. Stir in the flour, water, kimchi brine, rice vinegar, soy sauce, chopped kimchi, red bell pepper, sesame seeds, and salt until just combined. If needed, stir in 1 more tablespoon of water at a time until a thick but pourable consistency is achieved.

Allow the batter to rest for 5 minutes.

Warm 1 tablespoon of the oil in your largest skillet over medium-high heat.

Pour the batter in ¼-cup additions, 2 or 3 at a time in the skillet, to make 8 pancakes total. Cook for 2 to 3 minutes, until golden brown, then flip and cook for an additional 2 to 3 minutes.

Repeat with the remaining oil and batter until all the pancakes are cooked.

Meanwhile, make the dipping sauce by whisking the soy sauce, vinegar, honey, and sesame seeds together in a medium bowl.

Serve the pancakes with the dipping sauce.

NUTRITIONAL STATS PER SERVING (2 PANCAKES): 258 Calories, 7g Protein, 37g Carbohydrates, 9g Fat (1.5g Saturated), 44mg Cholesterol, 6g Sugars, 2g Fiber, 734mg Sodium

TOP NUTRIENTS: Vitamin C = 39%, Folate = 23%, Vitamin B1 = 19%, Iron = 17%, Vitamin B12 = 13%

Brainfood Reuben

MAKES 1 SANDWICH

Yes, you can make a probiotic grilled cheese "Reuben." Fermented cabbage and sourdough bread add a dose of good bugs to this rainy-day favorite. Pair with a simple salad or the Miso Butternut Squash Soup on page 226. Adding mayo is a great trick for toasting sandwiches. No extra oil or butter needed—just put the mayo-coated sandwich into a dry skillet.

2 slices thick-cut bacon

1 tablespoon mayonnaise

2 slices sourdough bread

1 ounce mozzarella cheese, grated

1/3 cup finely chopped sauerkraut

1/3 cup packed baby arugula

2 ounces white cheddar cheese, grated

Preheat the oven to 400°F.

Place the bacon on a parchment-lined rimmed baking sheet. Bake for 15 to 18 minutes, until crisp to your liking. Transfer to a paper towel to drain.

Heat a medium skillet over medium-low heat.

Spread the mayonnaise on both sides of the slices of bread, then place them on a cutting board. Mound the mozzarella on one side. Squeeze any excess liquid out of the chopped sauerkraut, then pile it on top of the mozzarella. Add the bacon slices, breaking them up as needed to cover the sandwich, then the arugula, then add the cheddar cheese and close the sandwich.

Add the sandwich to the heated skillet, press down gently with a spatula, and cook for 5 to 7 minutes, until golden brown. Carefully flip and cook for another 5 to 7 minutes, until golden brown on the second side.

Transfer the sandwich to a cutting board, let it rest for a couple minutes, then slice it in half.

NUTRITIONAL STATS PER SERVING: 721 Calories, 49g Protein, 55g Carbohydrates, 37.5g Fat (17g Saturated), 122mg Cholesterol, 5g Sugars, 4g Fiber, 1643mg Sodium

TOP NUTRIENTS: Selenium = 126%, Thiamine = 64%, Vitamin B12 = 50% Folate = 43%, Iron = 28%

REVIEW

Consider the following questions before you move on to Week 6:

1. Did you meet your goal of adding 3 to 5 servings of fermented foods this week?
2. Celebrate your successes! What approaches worked in helping you achieve that goal? What strategies could help as you move into next week?
3. Did you try any recipes? What skill could you work on to make it easier to add more of these foods to your meals next time?
4. How can you best continue to add fermented foods to your meals as you move forward?

GOOD MICROBIOME BUGS

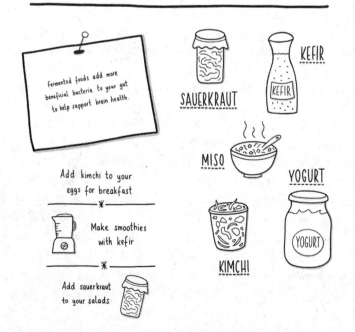

Fermented foods add more beneficial bacteria to your gut to help support brain health.

SAUERKRAUT

KEFIR

MISO

YOGURT

KIMCHI

Add kimchi to your eggs for breakfast

Make smoothies with kefir

Add sauerkraut to your salads

WEEK 6: GROWING YOUR FOOD ROOTS

While each and every one of us approaches food from a different perspective, one thing many of us have in common is that we're becoming increasingly removed from our food roots. We go to the grocery store and pick up prepackaged foods without a thought about where they come from or how we might better connect to our local food system and community at large. As you master eating to beat depression and anxiety, it's important to find ways to make those connections—whether it's hosting regular potluck meals, volunteering at your local farmers market, or investing in a community supported agricultural (CSA) share to get hold of fresh veggies. Your food roots—and the consequent strong connections you make with those around you—are just as important to your mental health as are the nutrients you consume.

Human beings are social by nature. It's not surprising that isolation and loneliness greatly increase the risk of depression and decrease the length and quality of our lives. Being part of a community that helps bring joy and pleasure to food is a key part of nourishing your brain and mental health long after you've completed the six-week plan. That's why I've asked that each week you engage in **one intentional action** to build your food connections and grow your food roots.

Over the years, I've felt my food roots grow as I've engaged with food communities all around the country and connected to the soil, farms, and people that create our web of nourishment. For me, it started when my parents moved back to the farm, but each step of my journey as an eater, from the food co-op at my college to the Abingdon Square Greenmarket in New York City where I rekindled my relationship with kale and farm-fresh produce, has helped solidify my mental health with a strong sense of interconnectedness.

How to Start

In what ways are you already connected to your food community? Who are the people and what are the local organizations involved? Does your community have a food co-op or farmers market? Do you have access to a CSA or community garden? What activities or community events leave you personally satisfied and connected?

Tips and Tricks

Roots grow strong and deep over time. Be patient, especially if you are still in the process of discovering the markets and co-ops around you—and, until now, your experience with food may have been more focused on efficiency than deepening your relationship with your local food community. Checking out your local farmers market is a great way to stock up while socializing with local growers and purveyors. Start with a small box or share of a CSA if you're adapting to eating more produce. Get to know your fishmonger and butcher. Ask them what's special at their counter. Check if a local farm has a volunteer day. Sign up for a cooking class at a neighborhood restaurant or school. Volunteer with your church to help with the food pantry. There are many creative ways to enhance your relationship with your food community—and become a more knowledgeable and confident eater in the process.

Challenges

Exploring new groups and experiences can be anxiety provoking, especially when we're not feeling our best. Building this personal food community can seem like an idealistic and overwhelming task if we don't focus on the simple, small acts that build it day by day, week by week. Like incorporating more nutrient-dense foods into your weekly diet, it all begins meal by meal, bite by bite. Don't make it more complicated than it needs to be. Remember, more dinner parties and potlucks are signs of progress.

REVIEW AND THE FUTURE

1. Did you meet your goal for the week of engaging in one intentional act to grow your food roots?
2. Celebrate your successes! What approaches worked in helping you achieve that goal? What strategies could help as you move into next week?
3. Did you share any recipes or notable meals with anyone?
4. How can you best continue to grow your food roots and deepen your sense of connectedness to your food community?

YOUR FOOD ROOTS

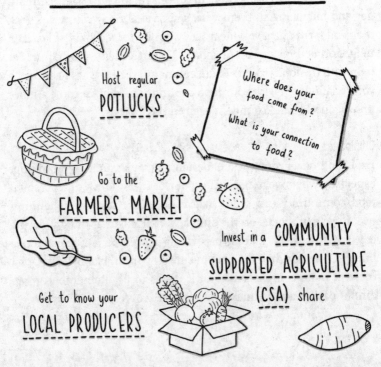

Host regular POTLUCKS

Where does your food come from?

What is your connection to food?

Go to the FARMERS MARKET

Invest in a COMMUNITY SUPPORTED AGRICULTURE (CSA) share

Get to know your LOCAL PRODUCERS

A STRONG FOUNDATION FOR GROWTH

I've mentioned before that how I treat depression and anxiety has radically changed over the last ten years. And the results have been phenomenal. Food really is medicine. And as you complete the six-week plan, I hope you've felt these same positive changes, not only with an improvement in your mood or anxiety levels but also with a boost of confidence. You now have a powerful set of tools to help you better care for your body, brain, and mental health. This plan was created to help you understand that brain health really does start at the end of your fork—and by incorporating the nutrient-dense foods that Mother Nature designed to feed your brain, you now have an action plan to continue that journey for the rest of your life.

Never forget that you have an opportunity every time you sit down to eat to put your brain into "grow" mode, to feed your microbiome, and to foster optimal brain health. As you continue to eat more nutrient-dense foods, you'll continue to feel better, not only because your brain has the building blocks it needs to work at its best but also because you know you're intentionally supporting your health and well-being. You have the knowledge and confidence you need to be a true master of self-nourishment.

One year from now and then in another decade, I hope you will look back over this plan and understand why eating with your brain in mind is so vital to mental health. By feeding your brain, you're protecting your most important asset. You now know the science behind diet. You've spent time better understanding your strengths when it comes to eating—and some challenges you may continue to face. You've worked through the six food categories to gain the expertise you need to eat with joy and purpose. You have all the tools you need to succeed as you eat to beat depression and anxiety, nurturing your mind, body, and spirit as you sit down to every meal.

FINAL REVIEW

Consider the following questions:

1. How do you feel now that you've completed the six-week plan?
2. Did you meet your goals?
3. Celebrate your successes! What approaches worked in helping you to better connect with your food roots? What didn't work as well?
4. Did you try any recipes? What skills could you work on to help make some of these dishes easier?
5. How can you reach out and build stronger connections with your greater food community?
6. How can you best continue to add nutrient-dense foods to your diet in a way that's nourishing to body, mind, and spirit?

CHAPTER 9: Recap

- Each week's section of the six-week plan addresses a specific food category to add to your diet: leafy greens; rainbows; seafood; nuts, beans, and seeds; good microbiome bugs; and your food roots.
- At the beginning and end of each week in the plan, consider how you can add the recommended number of servings of that particular food category to your meals. What are some easy ways to start? What challenges might you face? What SMART goals can you develop to help? Where might you improve?
- At the end of the six weeks, take stock of what you've accomplished. What approaches worked in helping you to add more nutrients to your meals? How can you best continue to do so in ways that nourish your body, mind, and spirit?

ACKNOWLEDGMENTS

I would like to thank my patients, current and past, who have taught me the most about mental health. It is a great honor to care for you. I would like to acknowledge the many researchers and scholars around the world who have contributed to the scientific foundation of this book. Good science concerning mental health and nutrition is very hard to do. We are forever in your debt. There are many opinions about what to eat, but it seems for the first time there is growing consensus that our food choices impact our mental health and brain health. I am especially grateful to Felice Jacka for her leadership; John Cryan and Robert McIntyre for their interviews; and the many researchers cited in the notes. Thank you, Laura LaChance, for all your work creating the Antidepressant Food Scale with me, and Emily Deans, for your friendship, thinking about nutrition, and writing for the public. I'm grateful to **all** my colleageus interested in Nutritional Psychiatry, especially Capt. Joseph Hibbeln, Phil Muskin, Georgia Edes, Lisa Masconi, and Uma Naidoo.

My work using food in mental health has grown exponentially in the last few years. I've traveled widely lecturing and conducting workshops around the country, supported by a small yet mighty team. Thank you, Samantha Elkrief, MSW, for your kindness, clinical skills, and friendship. Thank you, Andrew Luer, Xiaojue Hu, and Jennie West for our work together and for all of your support of me personally.

Thank you, Karen Rinaldi, for publishing my books, believing in the power of food is medicine, and sharing a good wave. Thank you, Haley Swanson, for your sharp edits and to Rebecca Raskin, Leda, Penny, Sophia, and the entire HarperWave team for all your efforts to make this book a reality and a success.

Thank you, Caroline Chambers, for developing the recipes for the book and Christine Locascio and Lindy Speakman for your help with the nutritional data. Thank you, Kayt Sukel, for all of your help making this book what it is. Katrin Wietek and I met on Instagram when she posted a sketch of a podcast I was on. It was whimsical, informative, and effective, a combo I adore. Since then, Katrin has created dozens of sketches about brain health and nutrition, many of which were created for this book. Cheers to your creativity.

My agent, Joy Tutela, and the David Black Agency have supported and pushed me. Thank you for always having your eyes on the prize.

I'd like to acknowledge the therapists and friends who have helped me with my mental health over the years and especially my psychoanalyst, Ron Puddu. Thanks for being a consummate clinician.

My professional colleagues in mental health have been incredibly supportive of my work. Thank you to my colleagues at Columbia Psychiatry, especially Lloyd Sederer, Deborah Cabaniss, and our chairman Jeff Lieberman. Working with the American Psychiatric Association Council on Communications has been an honor. Thank you to my colleagues on the council for all you do. This book came to life as several of my colleagues and friends took big steps. I've been inspired by many of the creative mental health clinicians making content, particularly Greg Scott Brown, Pooja Lakshmin, and Jessi Gold, all now writing up a storm. I am so encouraged by you and incredibly proud of what you do.

Nothing develops in isolation. I am indebted to the many media outlets that encourage my work. I greatly enjoy the creative process and learning more about modern media with each project.

Thank you to Rich Dorment, Spencer Dukoff, Marty Muson, Nojan Aminosharei, and the team at *Men's Health*, where I serve as an advisor. Thank you to my Medscape family, especially my editor Bret Stetka, John Rodriguez, and Liz Neporent. I've been very fortunate for wise counsel and support of many of the major players in the wellness space: Melisse Gelula, Mark Hyman, Dhru Purohit, Jason and Colleen Wacob, Chef David Bouley, Jim Gordon, Kathie Swift, and the Center for Mind Body Medicine; The Omega Institute, Kripalu, and TEDx, to name a few. Thank you, Maria Shriver, Annie Fenn, and the Women's Alzheimer's Movement. I am encouraged and inspired by the growing momentum to address mental health and fight stigma. Thank you all for keeping wind in the sails of innovation for mental health, wellness, and fitness.

Thank you, Marcia Lux, and Jerret, Emmet, and Hanna Matter for all the good times, Ian McSpadden for your brotherhood, and Dan Chrzanowski for your friendship and workouts. Thank you to my NYC crew. We'll meet again someday. We have been blessed in rural Crawford County, Indiana, with a caring community, an abundance of nature, and a group of progressive homeschoolers: thank you to the McSpadden, Howard, and Timberlake families for all you do to educate our kids. Thank you to Nikola Alford and the Maelstrom Barn family for helping me find balance.

Finally, I'd like to acknowledge my family and the sacrifices they make for me and this work. Books are hard and they make authors neurotic, internally preoccupied, and distracted. This book was written during the COVID-19 pandemic while we were in quarantine on our family farm in Southern Indiana. Living with my parents, my wife, our two kids, and our flock of chickens gave me the space and strength to continue my work, both as a physician suddenly practicing by telemedicine and as a man in continual development. It is a bumpy ride at times, and I am grateful for your understanding and faith in me. Thank you, Lucy, for your fierceness, your laughter, your love of process, and unwavering support of me and my fantastical ideas. And thank you, Greta and Forrest for making sure I keep the best stuff in life prioritized. That's you two and the daily joy of sharing life with you. This is the first book I've written that you can actually read, and I hope it helps explain all the wild salmon, arugula, and beans on our dinner table and what's been on my mind these months. I love you.

RESOURCES

Eating to beat depression and anxiety is a lifelong endeavor. As you move forward making changes to your diet, there is always more to learn and new food to discover. One of the many benefits of the growing Food Is Medicine and Nutritional Psychiatry movements is the increasing list of qualified experts and noteworthy organizations.

This chapter is filled with additional resources that can help support you and many that I have found helpful in my journey to understand food and Nutritional Psychiatry. Below you'll find the groups and organizations I recommend to my patients that offer easy ways to connect to your food roots, learn more about new studies in Nutritional Psychology, and support your mental health as you continue on this journey. For more resources go to www.DrewRamseyMD.com.

FOOD RESOURCES

United States Department of Agriculture (https://www.usda.gov/). When you see the nutritional information on food packaging, or in a recipe, social media post, or expert commentary, that information is likely based on data and research from a USDA laboratory. The USDA website provides data about food and offers a detailed nutritional analysis of anything you might think of eating, easily searchable by food type, preparation style, and portion size.

Food Tank (https://foodtank.com/). This food-inspired think tank is building a global community of healthy, nourished eaters through programs that support sustainable agriculture and food system change.

The Savory Institute (https://savory.global/). Allan Savory, an ecologist, has inspired the regenerative agriculture and pasture-based movements. The Savory Institute has programs to connect farmers, brands, and consumers with regenerative practices.

The Land Institute (https://landinstitute.org/). This organization supports science-based research to develop more sustainable agricultural practices, including perennial grain crops and polyculture farming solutions. The Land Institute means a lot to me. As a young physician starting to research the connection between food and mental health, I traveled out to Salinas, Kansas, to meet with Wes Jackson, the founder of this amazing organization. I learned a lot.

Local Harvest (http://www.localharvest.org). Looking for assistance in locating your nearest farmers market or community supported agriculture (CSA) outfit? Local Harvest, a strong supporter of the local food movement, can help. This amazing resource connects people directly to local farming operations with a comprehensive directory, as well as a regular newsletter that can be sent directly to your email inbox.

The Environmental Working Group (https://www.ewg.org/). The EWG is a nonprofit organization with a mission of protecting human health and the environment. It is an excellent resource for explaining the big issues affecting farming and food—as well as how to avoid common pesticides and contaminants.

Monterey Bay Aquarium (https://www.montereybayaquarium.org/). You may be surprised to see an aquarium on this list—but this really is one of the most gorgeous sea-life attractions in the country. Its mission is to inspire ocean conservation efforts, and its Seafood Watch team is working hard to make seafood consumption more sustainable.

NUTRITIONAL PSYCHIATRY AND FOOD IS MEDICINE RESOURCES

Food and Mood Centre (https://foodandmoodcentre.com.au/). Based at Australia's Deakin University, the Food and Mood Centre, directed by Felice Jacka, is a multidisciplinary research institution that studies how the food we eat influences our brain, mood, and overall mental health. Its overarching goal is to develop nutrition-based interventions to better prevent and treat mental health conditions.

APC Microbiome Institute (https://apc.ucc.ie/). Formerly known as the Alimentary Pharmabiotic Centre, the APC Microbiome Institute, located at Ireland's University College Cork, is one of the world's leading centers of microbiome research. There, researchers including John Cryan investigate the microbiome and how it influences health and disease.

Weill-Cornell Alzheimer's Prevention Clinic (https://weillcornell.org/services /neurology/alzheimers-disease-memory-disorders-program/our-services /alzheimers-prevention-clinic). Alzheimer's disease, a progressive neuro-degenerative disorder that destroys the brain's memory centers, is diagnosed in millions of Americans each year. Scientists now understand that this disease starts decades before symptoms are observed. And at the Weill-Cornell Alzheimer's Prevention Clinic, clinicians and scientists are studying the use of nutrition-based approaches to prevent this debilitating disorder.

The Center for Mind-Body Medicine (https://cmbm.org/). The Center for Mind-Body Medicine, based in Washington, D.C., works to promote evidence-based approaches to wellness. Its research programs work with the goal of creating practical, scientifically sound skills for self-care, nutrition, and self-awareness. Its work has highlighted the link between good nutrition and mental health.

Mark Hyman, MD (https://www.drhyman.com/). Mark Hyman is a leader in the Food Is Medicine movement. He is a practicing family physician and an internationally recognized leader, speaker, educator, and advocate in the field of Functional Medicine. He is the founder and director of the UltraWellness Center, the head of Strategy and Innovation of the Cleveland Clinic Center for Functional Medicine, and a thirteen-time *New York Times* bestselling author.

Rupy Aujla, MD (https://thedoctorskitchen.com). Dr. Rupy Aujla is a UK-based NHS physician making waves with his engaging content, delicious recipes, and top-ranked podcast.

Rebecca Katz, MS (https://www.rebeccakatz.com/). Rebecca Katz is culinary translator and chef well-known in the Food Is Medicine movement. An expert on how food can help sustain optimal health, she wrote *The Healthy Mind Cookbook*, which focuses on how nutrition can bolster physical and mental health.

The Brain Food Academy (https://the-brain-food-academy.teachable.com/). If you'd like more support as you learn to eat to beat depression and anxiety, my practice offers e-courses and other online resources at the Brain Food Academy.

MENTAL HEALTH RESOURCES

National Alliance on Mental Illness (https://nami.org/home). NAMI is the largest network of professionals working to provide advocacy, education, support, and public awareness of mental health conditions. It offers free groups and seminars, support for caregivers, and access to mental healthcare providers in your area.

American Psychiatric Association (https://www.psychiatry.org/). Full disclosure: I am a member, fellow, and past chairman of the Council on Communications for this incredible organization. The APA prides itself on its mission to ensure effective and accessible treatment for all people with mental health conditions, including substance use disorders.

Mental Health America (https://www.mhanational.org/). This community-based nonprofit organization helps to address the needs of individuals living with a mental health disorder. One of its big goals is work on prevention—and how we, as a country and society, can help our citizens prevent the development of mental illness.

National Institute of Mental Health (https://www.nimh.nih.gov/index .shtml). A key member of the National Institutes of Health (NIH), NIMH leads the federal charge on the study and treatment of mental disorders. The NIMH website is chock-full of information about different mental health disorders—and is a great resource for learning more about potential treatment options. I'd also add that NIMH's director, Joshua Gordon, is an incredible person and scientist. I know because I trained with him at Columbia University. He's the rare mix of top-notch research scientist, caring clinician, and capable institute administrator—and, under his direction, the institute is doing cutting-edge research on depression and anxiety.

American Foundation for Suicide Prevention (https://afsp.org/). The AFSP's mission is saving lives and bringing hope to those whose lives have been affected by suicide. It funds scientific research and educational programs, lobbies for public policy changes, and supports survivors of suicide loss.

Center for Motivation and Change (https://motivationandchange.com/). The CMC is a private group practice of clinicians and researchers in New York City who work to better understand and treat substance use and compulsive behaviors. Its treatment focus is on motivation—how to help patients find their own path toward change and overall well-being.

Substance Abuse and Mental Health Services Administration (https://www.samhsa.gov/). This federal agency, part of the U.S. Department of Health and Human Services, is responsible for public health efforts to promote behavioral and mental health. Its mission is to reduce the impact of mental health conditions, including substance abuse, across the country.

Overeaters Anonymous (https://oa.org/). This twelve-step program, modeled after the twelve steps of Alcoholics Anonymous, is a community program that supports people who suffer from compulsive eating and food behaviors.

David Puder, MD's Psychiatry and Psychotherapy Podcast (https://psychiatrypodcast.com/). This podcast, developed for mental health professionals and mental health enthusiasts, covers everything from how psychiatric medications work to the history of bipolar illness. If you are interested in learning more about mental health conditions—and the most common treatments for them—this is a great option.

Bring Change to Mind (https://bringchange2mind.org/). Cofounded by Oscar-nominated actress Glenn Close, this organization is working hard to end stigma and discrimination directed toward individuals suffering from a mental health condition.

Women's Alzheimer's Movement (https://thewomensalzheimersmovement.org/). This organization, founded by journalist Maria Shriver, is supporting research efforts to better understand why women are disproportionately affected by Alzheimer's disease. It offers educational programs to help people understand the link between sex and neurodegeneration and provides funding to innovative research projects trying to answer that very question.

NOTES

CHAPTER 1: THE NEW SCIENCE OF EATING FOR MENTAL HEALTH

1. D. S. Baldwin et al., "Efficacy of Drug Treatments for Generalized Anxiety Disorder: Systematic Review and Meta-Analysis," *British Medical Journal* 342 (2011): https://doi.org/10.1136/bmj.d1199.
2. J. C. Felger et al., "Inflammation Is Associated with Decreased Functional Connectivity within Corticostriatal Reward Circuitry in Depression," *Molecular Psychiatry* 21 (2016): 1358–65, https://www.nature.com/articles/mp2015168.
3. S. J. Leu et al., "Immune-Inflammatory Markers in Patients with Seasonal Affective Disorder: Effects of Light Therapy," *Journal of Affective Disorders* 63, no. 1–3 (2001): 27–34, https://www.sciencedirect.com/science/article/abs/pii/S0165032700001658.

CHAPTER 2: TWELVE NUTRIENTS FOR A BETTER BRAIN

1. A. Sánchez-Villegas et al., "Association of the Mediterranean Dietary Pattern with the Incidence of Depression: The Seguimiento Universidad de Navarra/University of Navarra Follow-up (SUN) cohort," *Arch Gen Psychiatry,* 66 no. 10 (October 2009): doi: 10.1001/archgenpsychiatry.2009.129.
2. C. T. McEvoy et al., "Neuroprotective Diets Are Associated with Better Cognitive Function: The Health and Retirement Study," *Journal of the American Geriatric Society* 65, no. 8 (2017): 1857–62, https://www.ncbi.nlm.nih.gov/pmc/articles/PMC5633651/.
3. P. Khanna et al., "Nutritional Aspects of Depression in Adolescents— A Systematic Review," *International Journal of Preventative Medicine* (April 3, 2019): doi: 10.4103/ijpvm.IJPVM_400_18, https://www.ncbi.nlm.nih.gov/pmc/articles/PMC6484557/.
4. H. M. Francis et al., "A Brief Diet Intervention Can Reduce Symptoms of Depression in Young Adults—A Randomized Controlled Trial,"

PLoS One (October 9, 2019): https://doi.org/10.1371/journal
.pone.0222768.

5. H. M. Francis et al., "A Brief Diet Intervention."

6. S. J. Torres et al., "Dietary Electrolytes Are Related to Mood," *British
Journal of Nutrition* 100, no. 5 (2008): 1038–45, https://www.ncbi
.nlm.nih.gov/pubmed/18466657.

CHAPTER 3: HOW TO GROW NEW BRAIN CELLS

1. M. Zhao et al., "BDNF Val66Met Polymorphism, Life Stress and
Depression: A Meta-Analysis of Gene-Environment Interaction,"
Journal of Affective Disorders 227 (2018): 226–35, https://www.ncbi
.nlm.nih.gov/pubmed/29102837.

2. J. C. Felger et al., "Inflammation Is Associated with Decreased
Functional Connectivity within Corticostriatal Reward Circuitry in
Depression," *Molecular Psychiatry* 21 (2016): 1358–65, https://www
.nature.com/articles/mp2015168.

3. G. Addolorato et al., "Anxiety but Not Depression Decreases in Coeliac
Patients after One-Year Gluten-Free Diet: A Longitudinal Study,"
Scandinavian Journal of Gastroenterology 36, no. 5 (2001): 502–06,
doi: 10.1080/00365520119754.

4. Y. Liao et al., "Efficacy of Omega-3 PUFAs in Depression: A Meta-
Analysis," *Translational Psychiatry* 9 (2019): 190, https://www.ncbi
.nlm.nih.gov/pmc/articles/PMC6683166/.

CHAPTER 4: OPTIMIZE YOUR GUT FOR MENTAL HEALTH

1. N. Sudo et al., "Postnatal Microbial Colonization Programs the
Hypothalamic-Pituitary-Adrenal System for Stress Response in Mice,"
Journal of Physiology 558, no. 1 (2004): 263–75, https://www.ncbi.nlm
.nih.gov/pubmed/15133062.

2. A. Madan et al., "The Gut Microbiota Is Associated with Psychiatric
Symptom Severity and Treatment Outcome among Individuals with
Serious Mental Illness," *Journal of Affective Disorders* 264 (2020):
98–106, https://www.sciencedirect.com/science/article/abs/pii
/S0165032719323523.

3. G. Winter et al., "Gut Microbiome and Depression: What We Know
and What We Need to Know," *Reviews in the Neurosciences* 29, no. 60
(August 28, 2018): 629–43, https://www.ncbi.nlm.nih.gov/pubmed
/29397391.

4. A. P. Allen et al., "*Bifidobacterium longum* 1714 as a Translational
Psychobiotic: Modulation of Stress, Electrophysiology, and

Neurocognition in Healthy Volunteers," *Translational Psychiatry* 6, no. 11 (November 1, 2016): e939, https://www.ncbi.nlm.nih.gov/pubmed/27801892.

5. H. Wang et al., "*Bifidobacterium longum* 1714 Strain Modulates Brain Activity of Healthy Brains during Social Stress," *American Journal of Gastroenterology* 114 (2019): 1152–62 doi: 10.14309/ajg.0000000000000203.

6. N. W. Bellano et al., "Enterochromaffin Cells Are Gut Chemosensors That Couple to Sensory Neural Pathways," *Cell* (2017): doi: 10.1016/j.cell.2017.05.034.

7. C. González-Arancibia et al., "Do Your Gut Microbes Affect Your Brain Dopamine?," *Psychopharmacology* 236, no. 5 (2019): 1611–22, https://www.ncbi.nlm.nih.gov/pubmed/31098656.

8. C. Fülling et al., "Gut Microbe to Brain Signaling: What Happens in Vagus . . . ," *Neuron* 101 (2019): 998–1002. https://doi.org/10.1016/j.neuron.2019.02.008

9. M. Pirbaglou et al., "Probiotic Supplementation Can Positive Affect Anxiety and Depressive Symptoms: A Systematic Review of Randomized Controlled Trials," *Nutrition Research* 36, no. 9 (2016): 889–98, https://www.ncbi.nlm.nih.gov/pubmed/27632908.

10. M. Pirbaglou et al., "Probiotic Supplementation."

CHAPTER 5: THE BEST FOODS TO BEAT DEPRESSION AND ANXIETY

1. C. Marques et al., "Gut Microbiota Modulation Accounts for the Neuroprotective Properties of Anthocyanins," *Scientific Reports* 8 (2018): 11341, https://doi.org/10.1038/s41598-018-29744-5.

2. S. E. Jackson et al., "Is There a Relationship Between Chocolate Consumption and Symptoms of Depression? A Cross-Sectional Survey of 13,626 US Adults." *Depress Anxiety* 36, no. 10 (2019): 987–95, https://doi.org/10.1002/da.22950.

3. A. M. Brickman et al. "Enhancing Dentate Gyrus Function with Dietary Flavanols Improves Cognition in Older Adults," *Nature Neuroscience* 17, no. 12 (2014): 1798–1803.

4. C. Tsang et al. "Effect of Polyphenol-Rich Dark Chocolate on Salivary Cortisol and Mood in Adults," *Antioxidants* 8, no. 6 (2019): 149, https://doi.org/10.3390/antiox8060149.

CHAPTER 6: CHALLENGES FACING THE MODERN EATER

1. K. E. Bradbury, N. Murphy, and T. J. Key, "Diet and Colorectal Cancer in UK Biobank: A Prospective Study," *International Journal of*

Epidemiology 49, no. 1 (February 2019): 246–58, https://academic
.oup.com/ije/advance-article/doi/10.1093/ije/dyz064/5470096.

2. S. Takenaka et al., "Feeding Dried Purple Laver (Nori) to Vitamin B12–
    Deficient Rats Significantly Improves Vitamin B12 Status," *British
    Journal of Nutrition* 85, no. 6 (2001): 699–703, doi: 10.1079
    /bjn2001352.

3. F. Watanabe et al., "Vitamin B12–Containing Plant Food Sources
    for Vegetarians," *Nutrients* 6, no. 5 (2014): 1861–73, https://doi.org
    /10.3390/nu6051861.

4. "Added Sugar in the Diet," *The Nutrition Source*, Harvard T.H. Chan
    School of Public Health, https://www.hsph.harvard.edu
    /nutritionsource/carbohydrates/added-sugar-in-the-diet/.

5. A. Knüppel et al., "Sugar Intake from Sweet Food and Beverages,
    Common Mental Disorder and Depression: Prospective Findings
    from the Whitehall II Study," *Scientific Reports* 7, no. 6287 (2017):
    https://www.nature.com/articles/s41598-017-05649-7.

CHAPTER 7: EATER, HEAL THYSELF

1. G. T. Doran, "There's a S.M.A.R.T. Way to Write Managements'
    Goals and Objectives," *Management Review* 70 (1981): 35–36.

CHAPTER 9: THE SIX WEEK PLAN AND RECIPES

1. Nutritional values were calculated using USDA data and percentages
    are based on the Dietary Reference Goals for women aged 31-50.
    The United States does not have an established recommendation
    for omega-3 fats. 500mg per day of combined EPA+DHA was used
    in the same method as employed in Eat Complete and based on
    international recommendations. For more information on Dietary
    Reference Goals see: https://health.gov/our-work/food-nutrition
    /2015-2020-dietary-guidelines/guidelines/appendix-7/.

INDEX

acetylcholine, 49, 50
almonds, 14, 51, 64–65, 75–76, 106, 183, 213, 221, 226
alpha-linolenic acid (ALA), 37–38
Alzheimer's disease, 166
amaranth, 134, 161
amino acids, 22, 34, 65, 88
anchovies, 14, 37, 105, 125, 180–81, 183, 203
anhedonia, 12
anthocyanins, 65, 75–76, 103–4, 191
anti-anxiety medications, 10
Antidepressant Food Scale (AFS), 13, 17, 32–33, 53, 74, 75, 99, 126
antidepressant medications, 10, 27, 29, 56, 69–70
anti-inflammatory drugs, 69–70
   anti-inflammatory molecules and foods, 12, 15
   anthocyanins, 65, 75–76, 103–4, 191
   coconut oil, 166
   flavonoids, 103–4, 193
   herbs and spices, 163, 164, 216
   imbalance with pro-inflammatory molecules, 67
   whole foods diet and, 72
antioxidants. See also vitamin A; vitamin C
   in black pepper, 164
   lycopene, 43, 103, 104, 121, 192
   rainbow fruits and vegetables and, 72, 103, 193

selenium and, 14, 41–42
   teas and, 133
anxiety, 9–10, 16
   caffeine and, 133
   celiac disease and, 72–73
   choline and, 49–50, 161
   essential nutrients to beat, 13–15, 34–52
   GI issues and, 77–78, 92
   inflammation and, 12, 67–69, 72–73, 76
   microbiome and, 52, 84, 89, 94
   new science of, 20–21
   nutrition and treatment of, 4, 6–7, 11, 17, 74–75
   omega-3s and, 38, 49
   probiotics treatment and, 90–91
   relationship with food and, 143
   SMILES study and, 31
   vitamins and minerals and, 14, 35, 42, 45, 48, 49
anxiety disorders, 23, 59, 61, 68, 71–72. See also generalized anxiety disorder
apple vs. apple juice, 93
artificial sweeteners, 131
arugula, 99, 102, 177, 178, 182, 186, 208, 230
asparagus, 35, 163, 199
asthma, 66
astrocytes, 66
autoimmune diseases, 66, 72–73, 133

Avocado Crema, 208–9
avocado oil, 187, 208, 215–16, 229
avocados, 74, 103, 104, 105, 183,
    184–85, 207
Avocado Toast, Crunchy Seedy, 195

bacteria. *See also* good microbiome
    bugs; probiotics
  in fermented foods, 108, 231
  in the gut, 51–52
  mediation of brain health and, 15,
    51–52, 80–84, 88–89, 94
  pathogenic, on greens, 178
  stress response and, 84–88, 92, 94
bananas
  for carb craving, 132
  in recipes, 176, 215–16, 224, 225,
    226
  nutrients in, 14, 40, 45, 215
barley, 133, 199
  basil, 162, 185–88, 190–91, 196,
    197, 200–201, 210–11, 217
batch cooking, 135, 168, 171, 217–18
BDNF. *See* brain-derived
  neurotrophic factor (BDNF)
beans. 45, 161-63, 214.
    See also legumes; nuts, beans,
    and seeds; *specific beans*
  dried, 161–62, 219
  fiber in, 93, 105, 109–10, 189, 213,
    221
  good microbiome bugs and,
    109–10
  in recipes, 183, 213, 216–17,
    217–18, 219, 226
beef, 14, 48, 50, 51, 107, 126
beets and beet greens, 40, 102, 182,
    186, 190
befriending protocols, 29–30
bell peppers, 47, 103, 104, 193, 199,
    207, 216–17, 229
beriberi, 43–44

Berk, Michael, 29
Berra, Yogi, 153, 154
berries. 103, 166–67 193.
    See also specific berries
  as sweetener, 104, 132, 161, 223
  BDNF and, 63, 65
  microbiome and, 92
  phytonutrients in, 65, 75–76,
    103–5, 225
  in recipes, 176, 182, 224, 225–26
bifidobacterium, 83–84, 85, 86–88,
    90, 92
bipolar disorder, 90
black beans, 106, 183, 219, 221
black pepper, 164, 165. *See also*
    within recipes
blenders, 156, 158–59
blood sugar, 42, 93
blueberries, 98–99, 104, 166, 191,
    224, 226
body fat reduction, 51
bok choy, 190–91, 198–99, 209
bonito flakes, 209–10
brain, 5-6
  atrophy/shrinkage of, 46, 58, 59,
    61
  composition and requirements of,
    19–23, 38, 53
  development of, 14, 34, 38, 53, 67,
    84–85
  energy needs of, 42, 43–44, 53, 166
  in grow mode, 58–61, 75, 102
  gut-brain axis, 78–79, 82, 89
  inflammation and, 66–69, 74
  magnesium and growth of, 38
  microbiome mediation of health of,
    15, 51–52, 80–84, 88–89, 94
  signaling in, 14–15, 42
brain cells, 38
  antioxidants and, 41–42
  building/development of, 37, 38,
    50–51, 166

growing new, 55–76
myelination (insulation) of, 14–15, 45–46, 49, 51
brain-derived neurotrophic factor (BDNF)
berries and, 63, 65
growing new brain cells and, 61–65
leafy greens and, 64
long-chain PUFAs and, 202
Mediterranean diet and, 64–65
microbiome and, 83
nuts and, 63, 64–65, 75–76, 106
omega-3 fats and, 37, 65, 75–76
seafood and, 63, 65, 75–76
turmeric and, 165
brain diseases and disorders, 24, 25, 26, 38
brain fog, 36, 42, 44, 91, 104, 111–12
Brain Food Clinic, 139–40, 173
brain food salad (general formula), 182–83
brain health, 12, 49
clinical randomized controlled trials and, 29–32
intersection of food and, 25–29
nutritional psychiatry and, 3–8, 16, 17
red meat and, 127
Brazil nuts, 14, 41, 180–81, 185, 221, 225
bread, 134, 195, 230
breast milk, human, 51
broccoli, 14, 47, 99, 103, 167, 193
brown rice, 132, 160, 199, 227
brussels sprouts, 13, 35, 47, 50, 99, 167, 194
buckwheat and buckwheat flour, 134, 215–16
Buckwheat Cacao Pancakes with Raspberry Compote, 215–16

butter, 129, 166, 210–11, 215–16, 218, 227–28. *See also* dairy products
butternut squash, 163
Butternut Squash Soup, Miso, 226–27
B vitamins. *See also* choline; *specific B vitamins*
bacteria and, 81, 82
in beans and legumes, 161, 219
brain health and, 22, 49
folate in, 13
green shakshuka and, 179
inflammation and, 76
in meat, eggs, and dairy category, 7, 106, 107–8, 109, 128

cabbage, 103, 124, 178, 198–99. *See also* kimchi; sauerkraut
cacao. *See also* dark chocolate
beans, 111, 112, 225
nibs, 111, 112, 215–16, 220, 225
powder, 225
Caesar, All Kale, 180–81
caffeine, 40, 133
calcium, 108, 120, 161, 176
Caldo Verde, 189
calories, 5, 107, 131, 134, 176, 214
cancer, 44, 48, 49, 66, 126
carbohydrate craving, brain food for, 132, 160, 196
carbohydrates, complex or slow-burning, 106, 131, 160, 161, 196, 197, 225–26
carbohydrates, simple or refined, 23, 26, 71, 72, 160. *See also* sugar
carcinogens, 24
cardiovascular disease, 16, 64
cardiovascular system, 165
carotenoids, 43, 44, 103, 107, 191–92, 193
carrots, 43, 182, 191–92, 193, 199, 209–10, 218

cashew butter, 220
Cashew-Caesar Dressing, 180–81
cashews, 105-6, 183, 184–85, 187,
   213, 221, 224, 226–27
Cassoulet, Mushroom and Chicken,
   217–18
cast-iron pans, 159
cauliflower, 103, 194
CBT (cognitive behavioral therapy),
   10
celiac disease, 72–73, 133
cell growth and division, regulation
   of, 43, 44
cellular waste disposal, 38, 40
Centers for Disease Control and
   Prevention, 98
cerebral spinal fluid (CSF), 47
ceviche, 203, 207, 212
Ceviche, Mango-Ginger Shrimp, 207
challenges to eating for mental
   health, 117–37
chard, 10, 99, 102, 178, 179, 199
cheddar cheese, 161, 187, 230
cheese, 129–30, 135, 161, 162,
   185–88. *See also* dairy products;
   specific cheeses
cherries, 15
chia seeds, 215–16, 220
chicken, 102, 107
   in recipes, 184, 190–91, 217–18
   herbs and spices and, 162, 163,
      164, 190–91
   nutrients in, 45, 128
chickpeas (garbanzo beans), 35, 45,
   99, 161, 183, 189, 219, 221
chiles, 15, 164, 195
chili powder, 164
chives, 161, 162, 199, 204, 205, 211
Chocolate Brain Truffles, 220
Chocolate Peanut Butter Cup
   Smoothie, 225
cholesterol, 13, 128, 129

choline, 7, 49–50, 107–8, 109,
   129, 161, 179, 209
cilantro, 162–63, 179, 186, 188, 196,
   199, 205-206, 207, 208–9
circulatory system, 164
Citrus Vinaigrette, 184
clams, 15, 46–47, 48, 125, 203
Clams, Simple Steamed, with Fresh
   Herbs and Lemon, 210–11
clinical randomized controlled
   trials, 28, 29–32, 46, 53
clinical remission, 31
cloves, 186
cobalamin. *See* vitamin B12
   (cobalamin)
Cobb Salad, Brain Food, 184–85
cocoa, 110, 111, 112
coconut milk or cream, 187, 216–17
Coconut-Ginger Lentil Soup, 216–17
coconut oil, 166, 208, 215–17, 226
cod, 105, 149, 208–9
cofactors, 47–48
coffee, 133
cognition, 52, 59, 85
cognitive behavioral therapy (CBT),
   10
colanders, 156, 157, 158
collard greens, 93, 96, 102, 178, 179,
   189, 199
community supported agriculture
   (CSA), 109, 135, 232, 233, 234
concentration, diminished, 8, 16,
   44–45, 111
cooking fats, 165–66, 208
cortex, 20, 83
cortisol, 9, 83, 86, 89, 111
c-reactive protein (CRP), 65, 68
crème fraîche, 204
Cryan, John, 79, 80, 84–87, 91–92
cumin, 164, 179, 219
curcumin, 165
curry, 164

cutting boards, 156, 157
cytokines, 65, 70, 74

dairy fats, 23–24, 129–30
dairy products
 fermented, 108, 109, 130, 222–23
 fat in, 108, 109
 grass-fed, 166
 inflammation and intolerance to,
  108
 vaccenic acid and, 51
 vitamins in, 44, 46–47
dark chocolate. 36, 63, 74, 110–12,
 161, 220, 223, 224. *See also* cacao
dashi, 203, 209–10
dementia, 25, 44
dentate gyrus, 110
 depression, 8–9, 16, 20–21
 celiac disease and, 72–73
 clinical randomized controlled
  trials and, 29–32
 nutrients to beat, 13–15, 34–52
 hippocampus and, 58, 59
 homocysteine and, 34
 inflammation and, 12, 68–70,
  72–73, 76
 Mediterranean diet and, 25–27,
  29–31
 microbiome and, 84, 94
 nutrition and treatment of, 4–6,
  10–11, 17, 74–75
 probiotics treatment and, 90–91
 red meat intake and, 127
 vagus nerve stimulation for
  treatment of, 89
diabetes, 16, 51
Diagnostic and Statistical Manual
 of Mental Disorders (DSM-5),
 8–9, 16
dietary coaching or intervention,
 27–28, 29–32, 64–65, 73, 92
dietary patterns, 145–47, 148, 149, 152

diet culture, 117–19
digestion, 81, 82, 83
dips and dipping sauces, 104, 194,
 229
DNA, 34, 35, 103, 193
DNA synthesis, 38, 41, 42
docosahexaenoic acid (DHA), 14,
 37–38, 43, 44, 46, 202
dopamine, 14, 22, 24, 35–36, 45,
 46, 89

eggplants, 104, 191, 193
eggs, 107–8, 109, 128–29, 161, 176,
 179, 231
 allergies to, 123
 in recipes, 180, 183–85, 185,
  199–201, 205–206, 209–10,
  215–16, 228
 choline and, 7, 50, 107–8, 129,
  209
 hard-boiled, 144, 183, 184–85
 vitamins in, 14, 44, 46–47
eggs and dairy food category, 107–9,
 114. *See also* dairy products; eggs
eicosapentaenoic acid (EPA), 14,
 37–38, 202
Elkrief, Samantha, 140, 147, 148,
 149, 151, 173
emotional (limbic) system, 58, 59
emotion and inflammation, 67, 74
Enck, Paul, 87–88
endocannabinoids, 22
endocrine system, 80, 82
 energy, 8, 14, 16, 34–36, 42–44,
  50, 111, 142
enterochromaffin cells, 88–89
environment, gene expression and,
 57, 75
environmental sustainability,
 106–7, 109, 126
environmental toxins. *See* toxins
enzyme function, 48

EPA (eicosapentaenoic acid), 14,
    37–38, 202
epicatechin, 110, 111
epigenetics, 57, 75
evolution and inflammation, 68, 69
exercise, 27, 42, 71
extra-virgin olive oil (EVOO), 166
extrinsic motivation, 148

farmers markets, 95–96, 130, 232,
    233, 234
farro, 197–98, 199, 227
fasting, intermittent, 131–32, 133
fat burning, 51
fatigue, 9, 16, 48, 134
fats, cooking, 165–66, 208. See also
    olive oil
fats, healthy, 25, 26
    in avocados, 104, 183
    in recipes, 183, 187
    in dairy products, 129, 166
    in grass-fed beef, 107, 127
    in nuts, beans, and seeds, 106,
        214
fear, 67, 68–69, 74
fennel, 199
fermented foods. See also good
    microbiome bugs; kimchi; miso;
    sauerkraut
    in recipes, 182, 198–99, 209–10
    dairy products, 108, 109, 130,
        222–23 (see also kefir; yogurt)
    good microbiome bugs and, 12,
        91–93, 94, 110
    live cultures in, 222, 223, 226
    sourdough, 134
feta cheese, 179, 183, 196–97
fetal development, 34
fiber
    brain health and, 15
    in recipes, 215, 225–26
    in dark chocolate, 111, 220

good microbiome bugs and, 91–93,
    94, 109–10, 176, 193, 222
inflammation and, 71
in leafy greens, 93, 98, 99, 102,
    103, 176, 178
in millet, 161
in mushrooms, 197, 217
in beans, nuts and seeds, 93, 105,
    109–10, 189, 213, 221
in rainbows, 104, 109–10, 191, 193
Fifty Shades of Kale (Ramsey), 95,
    96
fight-or-flight response, 9–10
fish, 13, 32, 105, 166, 169, 202, 203.
    See also specific fishes
    dislike of, 124–26
    fats and, 37, 51, 124
    herbs and spices added to, 162,
        163, 164
    iron and, 48
    smoked, 212
fish flakes, 209–10
fish tacos, 100, 132, 203, 212
Fish Tacos with Avocado Crema,
    208–9
flavanols and flavonoids 103–4, 110,
    111, 193, 220
flax seeds and meal, 37, 204, 215
flaxseed oil, 51
flours, 160, 215–16
fluoxetine (Prozac), 10, 70
flu symptoms, 67–68
focus, 35, 36, 50, 111
folate
    deficiency in, 24
    foods containing, 34, 98, 102, 107,
        128, 104, 144, 176, 177, 216
    good microbiome bugs and, 82
    as key nutrient, 13, 17, 34–35
    serotonin and, 22
food allergies and sensitivities, 101,
    123, 133–34, 220

Food and Mood Centre, 29, 59, 127, 242–43
Food as Medicine movement and resources, 3, 96, 242–44
food assessments, 140–41
food categories, 98-112, 114
food, intersection with brain health, 25–29, 53
food journaling, 145–47, 152
food landscape, changing, 23–25
food, relationship with, 143–45, 151, 152
food resources, 241–42
food roots, growing, 232–34
foxtail millet, 161
Francis, Heather, 31–32, 106
free radicals, 15, 41, 72
Fried Rice with Peanut Sauce, Brainbow Kimchi, 198–99
frozen foods, 166–67, 193, 226
fruits, 25, 40, 71, 143–44, 166–67, 224, 225–26. *See also* rainbows; *specific fruits*

garlic, 124, 163, 177, 205, 206. *See also within recipes*
garlic powder and garlic salt, 164–65, 180–81, 184, 205, 208–9
gastrectomy, 79
gastrointestinal (GI) tract, 77–94. *See also* microbiome
  celiac disease and gluten sensitivity and, 133, 134
  gut-brain axis, 78–79, 82
  microbiome mediation of brain health, 15, 51–52, 80–84, 88–89, 94
gene expression, 57, 75
generalized anxiety disorder, 9, 11, 16
genetics, 21, 55–57, 75
germ-free animals, 81–83

ghee, 166
ginger, 125, 199, 205, 206, 207, 216–17
glial cells, 20–21, 22, 66
glucose, 42, 43, 93
glutamate, 22, 49, 89
glutathione, 41, 42
gluten, 72–73, 133–34
gluten-free flour, 215
goals for success, 149–51, 152
goat cheese, 130, 183
Gomez-Pinella, Fernando, 59–60
good microbiome bugs, 12, 13, 51–52, 109–10, 176, 193, 222–31. *See also* microbiome; fermented foods
grains, 133–34, 160–61. *See also* whole grains
Grain Salad, Roasted Shiitake and Spinach, 197–98
grapefruit and grapefruit juice, 163, 184–85, 207
grapeseed oil, 208
grass-fed animal products, 107, 108, 109, 127, 166, 215–16
graters, 156, 158
gut. *See* gastrointestinal (GI) tract
gut-brain axis, 78–79, 82, 89

halibut, 41
hazelnuts, 64, 75–76
heart disease and heart health, 13, 24–26, 34, 51, 126–27, 129, 165
heavy metal contaminants, 121, 125
hemoglobin, 13–14, 35, 36
hemp seeds, 37, 51, 220
herbs, 162–63. See also within recipes; specific herbs
hippocampus, 58, 59–60, 67, 75, 83
homeostasis, 41, 79
homocysteine, 34, 35, 44, 45, 46
honey, 132, 161, 199, 223, 225, 229

hormones, 21, 67, 89.
    See also specific hormones
hummus, 104, 164, 219
hydroxytyrosol, 165

immune system, 20, 48, 65–69, 80, 82, 89, 164
imperfect produce, 135–36
incomplete remission, 10
Indian cuisine, 164, 166
infections, 48, 49, 67–68
    inflammation, 13, 74, 76
    antioxidants and, 42, 44, 47
    brain function and, 4, 12, 66–69
    causes of, 71–73
    choline and, 49, 50
    chronic, 66, 68, 72
    dairy products and, 108
    depression and anxiety and, 12, 20, 68–70
    dietary interventions and, 92
    flavanols and, 111
    gluten sensitivity and, 134
    immune system and, 20, 65–66
    kynurenic acid and, 104
    fats and, 37, 38, 51, 107, 165, 202
    microbiome and, 71, 80, 81, 84–85, 226
    phytonutrients and, 50–51, 176, 193, 196, 216
    probiotics and, 90
    red meat and, 126
    vagus nerve and mediation of, 89
    vitamins and minerals and, 34, 35, 44, 45, 46, 48, 49
Instant Pots, 159, 160, 168
insulin sensitivity, 51
interest in activities, decreased, 8–9, 16, 67–68
interleukin-6, 65, 68
intrinsic motivation, 148
iodine, 41, 103

iron
    absorption of, 36, 48
    in cumin, 164
    in dark chocolate, 111
    deficiency in, 98
    in greens, 103, 128, 176
    as key nutrient, 13–14, 17, 35–36
    in meat, eggs, and dairy category, 106, 107, 109, 128
    in nuts, beans, and seeds, 105, 185, 189, 221
    in seafood, 105, 202, 212
    serotonin and, 22
irritability, 9, 16, 36, 42, 45, 67
irritable bowel syndrome (IBS), 77–78, 85, 92
Italian sausage, 189, 217

Jacka, Felice, 29–31, 33, 59–62, 92, 127, 135
junk foods, 122, 160

kale, 15, 40, 95–99 102–3, 167
    in recipes, 176, 179, 180–81, 182, 185–88, 189, 190–91, 224
    six week plan and, 175, 176, 178
Kale and Basil Pesto, 185–88
Kale Caesar, All, 180–81
Kefir, 108
    good microbiome bugs and, 93, 108, 110, 130, 222, 226, 231
    lactose intolerance and, 130
    in smoothies, 92, 132, 143–44, 176, 224, 225–26, 231
    sweeteners for, 104, 223
kefir dressing, 183
ketogenic diets, 101, 118, 132–33, 166
ketosis, 133, 166
kidney beans, 161, 219
kidneys, 121
kimchi, 110, 183, 198–99, 223, 228–29, 231

Kimchi Fried Rice with Peanut Sauce, Brainbow, 198–99
Kimchi Pancakes, 228–29
kitchen, 153–71
  contents of, organizing, 154–56, 170
  creating your workspace, 153–54, 170
  healthy staples and stores, 160–67, 170
  planning ahead, 168, 171
  shopping tips, 167
  shortcuts, 168–70, 171
  toolkit, building, 156, 157–59, 170
knives, 156, 157, 158
kombucha, 110, 222
kombu seaweed, 209–10
kynurenic acid, 104

LaChance, Laura, 13, 17, 32–33, 49, 53, 99
lactation, 45, 48
lactobacillus, 85, 89, 90, 92
lactose intolerance, 130
lard, 51
Lasagna, Turkey Zucchini Skillet, 200–201
leafy greens. 96, 97–98, 102. See also leaves; specific greens
  adding to diet, 7, 150
  affordability of, 134–35
  BDNF production and, 64
  dislike of, 123–24
  fiber and, 93, 102, 103, 176, 178
  folate and, 13, 34, 98, 102, 144, 176, 177
  as food category, 102–3, 114
  frozen, 167
  grains added to, 160, 161
  inflammation and, 72, 176
  magnesium and, 40, 178
  omega-3 fats and, 37

phytonutrients and, 102, 103, 176, 177, 178
  six week plan and recipes, 175–91
  in smoothies, 5, 102, 143–44, 150, 176, 225, 226
  washing, 178
learning and memory, 49–50, 51, 58, 110, 111, 129
leaves, 34, 41, 44, 48. See also leafy greens
  legumes, 14, 29, 34–36, 40, 92, 105–6, 135, 161–62. See also beans; nuts, beans, and seeds
lemons and lemon juice, 36, 48, 210–11. See also within recipes
lentils, 35, 93, 105–6, 161, 164, 216–17, 221
Lentil Soup, Coconut-Ginger, 216–17
lettuce, 7, 118, 124, 143, 177, 182
lifestyle, 10, 21, 29, 57
lifestyle intervention study, 27–28
limbic (emotional) system, 58, 59
limes and lime juice, 186, 188, 199, 206, 207, 208–9, 226
lipid synthesis, 49
liver (as food), 13, 14, 15, 35, 43, 46, 50, 107
liver, human, 46, 121
lobster, 41, 125
local farms and farmers, 107, 109, 127, 232, 233, 234
long-chain omega-3 fatty acids, 14, 17, 37–38, 105, 124, 202, 204, 205, 212
long-chain polyunsaturated fats (PUFAs), 37–38, 202
low-fat diet, 64
lutein, 43
lycopene, 43, 103, 104, 121, 192

macadamia nuts, 187
mackerel, 14, 125

magnesium
  brain health and, 22
  in dark chocolate, 111
  deficiency in, 24
  inflammation and, 74, 76
  as key nutrient, 14, 17, 38–40
  in leafy greens, 40, 178
  in meat, eggs, and dairy category,
    109, 128
  in millet, 161
  in nuts, beans, and seeds, 185,
    187, 215, 217, 219, 221
  in supplements, 120, 121
mahi-mahi, 100
major depressive disorder, 8, 29, 46
mangoes, 166–67, 207, 224
Mango-Ginger Shrimp Ceviche, 207
maple syrup, 132, 215–16
margarine, 23–24
marinades, 163
mayonnaise, 187, 230
McIntyre, Roger, 67, 68, 69
MCTs (medium-chain triglycerides),
  166
meal prep kits, 169
meat. 106–7, 109, 114
    See also specific meats
  grass-fed, 51, 107, 109, 127
  herbs and spices and, 163, 164
  iron and, 36
  processed, 71, 72, 109, 126
  red meat and heart health, 126–27
  vaccenic acid and, 51
  vitamins in, 44, 45, 46, 47
Mediterranean diet
  BDNF production and, 64–65
  brain health and, 12–13
  dairy products in, 108
  depression and anxiety and, 17,
    25–27, 29–31, 32
  grow mode and, 58–61, 75
  inflammatory markers and, 72

  microbiome and, 92
  olive oil and, 51, 165
medium-chain triglycerides (MCTs),
  166
melatonin, 44
memory and learning, 49–50, 51,
  59, 110, 111, 129
mental fatigue, 41
mental health resources, 244–45
mercury, 105, 125, 203
metabolic syndrome, prevention of,
  51
metabolism, 41, 42
methylation cycle, 50
Mexican cuisine, 5, 100, 162
microbiome. *See also* bacteria; good
  microbiome bugs
  anthocyanins and, 104
  diversity of, 81, 84, 85, 89, 90, 92,
    94, 109
  fiber and, 176, 215
  inflammation and immune system
    and, 20, 71, 80, 81, 84–85, 226
  mediation of brain health by,
    4, 12–13, 15, 51–52, 80–84,
    88–89, 94
  probiotics treatment and, 90–94
microglia, 66, 67
microgreens, 195
micronutrient deficiencies, 98
microorganisms in the gut, 51–52,
  80, 82, 94. *See also* bacteria;
  good microbiome bugs
microplastics, 105, 125, 203
milk, 129–30, 215–16. *See also* dairy
  products
millet, 161
minerals. *See* vitamins and
  minerals
miso, 110, 185, 187, 222, 226–27, 231
Miso Butternut Squash Soup, 226–27
miso dressing, 183

monounsaturated fatty acids
    (MUFAs), 51, 104, 127, 161, 165,
    195
mood
    choline and, 50
    dark chocolate and, 111–12
    depression and, 8, 16
    gluten sensitivity and, 134
    gut bacteria and, 52, 91
    hippocampus growth and, 58
    inflammation and, 67
    kynurenic acid and, 104
    regulation of, 14, 22, 46
    vitamins and minerals and, 34,
        35, 36, 38–39, 41, 44, 46
mood disorders, 23, 59, 61, 69,
    71–72
motivations, 148–59
mozzarella cheese, 200–201, 230
MUFAs, 51, 104, 127, 161, 165, 195
multivitamin supplements, 33,
    120–21
muscle building, 51, 166
Mushroom and Chicken Cassoulet,
    217–18
mushrooms, 14, 162–63, 217–18
mussels, 15, 46–47, 105, 125, 202,
    203, 212
mustard, 51, 180–81, 184, 227–28
mustard greens, 15, 43, 175, 176
myelin and myelination of brain
    cells, 14–15, 35, 36, 45–46, 49,
    51, 129
myoglobin, 35

navy beans, 93
nervonic acid, 51
nervous system, 44, 88–89, 165
neural circuit and neural network
    activity, 67
neural signaling, 40–41, 47–48
neurogenesis, 50–51, 59

neuromuscular conduction, 38
neurons (nerve cells)
    brain function and, 19–21, 53
    damaged, 66, 67
    in GI tract, 78, 80, 82, 88–89
    potassium and, 14, 40–41
neuroplasticity
    nutrients and, 11–12, 13, 14, 15, 37,
        44, 49
    epigenetics and, 57
    grow mode and, 58, 61
neuroprotectins, 38
neurotransmitters. See also specific
        neurotransmitters
    nutrients and, 5-6, 34, 35–36, 44,
        49, 129
    depression and anxiety disorders
        and, 21–22
    release into nervous system,
        88–89
neurotrophins, 60, 61–62, 72
nonsteroidal anti-inflammatory
    drugs (NSAIDs), 69–70
norepinephrine, 14, 44, 45
nut butters, 199, 220
nutrient-dense foods, 7, 15–16, 22,
    49, 75, 96, 174
nutritional psychiatry, 3–8, 16, 21,
    242–44
nuts. 25, 32, 105–6, 135, 214.
    See also nuts, beans, and seeds;
    specific nuts
    added to yogurt, 132
    allergies to, 123
    BDNF production and, 63, 64–65,
        75–76, 106
    in bread, 134
    fat and calorie content of, 214
    fiber and, 93, 105, 213, 221
    in recipes, 176, 183, 185–88, 213,
        214, 224, 225–26
    as snacks, 5, 106, 213, 214, 221

nuts *(continued)*
  vitamins and minerals in, 14, 36, 40, 49
  nuts, beans, and seeds. 105–6, 114, 213-22. *See also* beans; legumes; nuts; seeds

oats/oatmeal, 14, 134, 161, 220
obesity, 71
oleic acid, 51, 221
oleoylethanolamide, 51
olive oil. *See also within recipes*
  in brain food salad, 183
  on gnocchi, 132
  Mediterranean diet and, 25, 27, 29, 32, 64, 75
  MUFAs in, 51
  in sauce with garlic, 163
  as staple, 165–66
  synergism with other nutrients, 121
omega-3 fats. *See also* long-chain omega-3 fatty acids
  BDNF production and, 65, 75–76
  brain health and, 22, 49
  in eggs, 128–29
  grass-fed beef and balance of, 107, 127
  hippocampus growth and, 58, 59
  inflammation and, 71, 72, 74, 76
  nutritional psychiatry and, 3–4
  overview of, 37–38
omega-6 fatty acids, 71, 107
onions, 92, 124, 132, 227–28.
    See also within recipes
oranges and orange juice, 13, 15, 184–85
oregano, 200, 218
oxidative damage and oxidative stress, 41, 131–32
oxygen, 13–14, 35, 36, 40–41, 44

oysters, 99, 105, 212
  BDNF production and, 65
  kosher diets and, 125
  lack of toxins in, 203
  long-chained omega-3 fats and, 14, 37
  vitamins and minerals and, 14, 15, 36, 46, 48, 105
oyster shuckers, 158

pain, chronic, 41
Pancakes, Buckwheat Cacao, with Raspberry Compote, 215–16
Pancakes, Kimchi, 228–29
papaya, 47
Parmesan cheese, 180–81, 185–88, 197–98, 200–201
parsley, 163, 184–85, 186, 190–91, 196, 211
pasta, 102, 134, 150, 160, 163, 178, 202
pasta cooking method for grains, 197
pastured-raised animals, 107, 109
peanuts and peanut butter, 187, 199, 220, 224, 225
peanut sauce, 198–99
peas, 42
pecans, 42, 187, 220
Pecorino Romano cheese, 187, 217–18
Pepita-Parmesan Crunch, 180–81
Pepita-Pecorino Breadcrumbs, 217–18
pepitas. *See* pumpkin seeds
peppers, 105, 182, 208, 199, 207, 216–17, 229. See also specific peppers
peptic ulcers, 79
personal psychology, 21
pesticides, 109
pesto, 144, 177, 178, 185–88

Pete, 4–6, 55–56, 74, 99–100, 142
phosphatidylcholine, 49, 50
photosynthesis, 39
phytonutrients
    absorption of, 121
    in berries, 225
    in grains, 160, 161
    in herbs and spices, 162, 163, 164
    inflammation and, 50–51, 76, 176,
        193, 196, 216
    in leafy greens/leaves, 98, 99,
        102, 103, 176, 177, 178
    in mushrooms, 197, 217
    in nuts, beans, and seeds, 213, 221
    in olive oil, 165–66
    in rainbows, 50–51, 103–4, 191,
        193, 196
    salmon burgers and, 205
    supplements and, 120–21
    whole foods and, 72
pine nuts, 185–88, 221
pistachios, 187, 188, 220
pleasure, 8–9, 12, 16, 34, 35
plums, 227–28
polyphenols, 111, 133, 161
polyunsaturated fatty acids, 125,
    128, 161
pomegranates, 166–67
pork, 14, 42, 227–28
Pork Chops, One-Skillet, with
    Plums and Red Onion, 227–28
potassium
    foods containing, 14, 40, 104, 111,
        164, 178
    as key nutrient, 17, 40–41
    in recipes, 204, 215, 217
potatoes, 45, 162–63, 189, 202, 204
Potato Pancakes with Smoked
    Salmon and Crème Fraîche, 204
potluck meals, 232, 233, 234
PREDIMED-NAVARRA trial, 64

pregnancy, 34, 42, 45, 48
preservatives, 23, 24, 53, 223
probiotics, 12, 81, 83–84, 86–88,
    94, 199
probiotic supplements, 90–91, 94
    processed foods. 23 24, 26, 91,
        122–123, 130, 160, 167. *See
        also* carbohydrates, simple or
        refined
    dairy products, 108
    meats, 71, 72, 109, 126
pro-inflammatory molecules
    depression and anxiety and,
        68–69, 70
    EPA and, 38
    GI tract and, 80, 88
    imbalance with anti-inflammatory
        molecules, 67
    nuts and protection from, 65
    omega-3 fatty acids and, 72
    phytonutrients and, 72, 103
    probiotic treatment and, 90
    processed foods and, 91
    whole foods diet and, 75
Prosciutto Chicken with Sautéed
    Greens, Herby, 190–91
protein
    in dark chocolate, 111
    in meat, eggs, and dairy products,
        7, 106, 107–8
    in miso, 226
    neurotransmitters and, 22
    in nuts, beans, and seeds, 106,
        189, 213, 216, 219
    in seafood, 105, 205
    in whole grains, 161
Prozac, 10, 70
psychobiotic diet, 91–92
The Psychobiotic Revolution (Cryan),
    79
psychotherapy, 10, 27, 28, 30

PUFAs, 37–38, 202
pumpkin, 43
pumpkin seeds. 105–6, 221.
   See also within recipes
   fiber in, 99
   minerals in, 14, 15, 36, 48, 65,
      74, 99
purple nori, 128
pyridoxine, 44

quinoa, 134, 161, 197–98

radishes, 195, 208, 209–10
rainbows (colorful fruits and
   vegetables)
   affordability of, 134–35
   Build the Rainbow exercise, 192
   cooking fats and, 165
   fiber in, 104, 109–10, 191, 193
   as food category, 103–5, 114
   good bugs and, 109–10
   grains added to, 160, 161
   herbs and spices added to, 162,
      163, 164
   inflammation and, 72
   phytonutrients and, 50–51, 103–4,
      191, 193, 196
   six week plan and recipes, 182,
      191–201
   vitamins and minerals in, 34, 40,
      41, 42, 44, 45, 48
raspberries, 93
Raspberry Compote, 215–16
Recommended Daily Allowance
   (RDA), 24
red blood cells, production of, 44
red grapes, 65
regenerative agriculture, 109
reproduction, 41
resolvins, 38
resveratrol, 65
retinol. See vitamin A

Reuben, Brainfood, 230
rheumatoid arthritis, 66
rice, 134, 160, 196, 198–99
rice cookers, 159, 160
romaine lettuce, 182, 184
rosemary, 163
rosmanol, 163
rosmarinic acid, 163
rumenic acid, 51
rye, 133

sage, 163
salad dressings, 162, 180–81, 184, 198
salads, 178, 180–85, 197–98, 221, 231
   salmon, 105, 212
   in fish tacos, 100
   frozen, 167
   nervonic acid in, 51
   rice added to, 160
   smoked, 183, 195, 202, 204
   wild, 14, 37, 46, 98–99 105,
      184–85, 204–206
Salmon Burgers, Wild, 205–6
sardines, 37, 100, 105, 125, 183, 203,
   212
sauerkraut, 92, 93, 110, 183, 222,
   227–28, 230, 231
sausage, Italian, 189, 217
scallops, 50
scurvy, 48
sea bass, 167
seafood. See also specific seafoods
   BDNF production and, 63, 65,
      75–76
   bivalves, 46–47, 105, 125, 210
   concerns about eating, 105,
      124–26, 203
   dislike of, 99–100
   as food category, 105, 114
   frozen, 167
   grow mode and, 75
   inflammation and, 71, 72, 74

learning to cook, 149
long-chained omega-3 fats and, 14, 37, 38
Mediterranean diet and, 25
six week plan and recipes, 183, 202–12
vitamins and minerals and, 36, 42, 44, 45, 46–47
seasonal affective disorder (SAD), 12
seaweed, 103, 128, 209–10
seeds, 105–6. *See also* nuts, beans, and seeds; *specific seeds*
  in bread, 134
  fiber and, 105, 213, 221
  minerals in, 36, 40, 49
  in recipes, 183, 185–88, 195, 196–97, 224, 225–26
selective serotonin reuptake inhibitors (SSRIs), 10, 61, 70
selenium, 14, 17, 22, 41–42, 105, 109, 128, 202, 212
Sequenced Treatment Alternatives to Relieve Depression (STAR*D), 10
serotonin
  dietary interventions and, 92
  neurons releasing, 88–89
  SSRIs and, 61, 70
  vitamins and minerals and, 14, 22, 34, 35–36, 41, 44, 45, 46, 49
sesame seeds, 36, 48, 187, 195, 196, 199, 209–10, 229
Shakshuka, Green, 179–80
shears, kitchen, 156, 158
sheet pan meals, 168
sheet pans, 156, 159
shellfish, 123. *See also specific shellfish*
shiitake mushrooms, 197–98
short-chained fatty acids, 81
shrimp, 41, 100, 125, 162, 167, 183, 184, 202
Shrimp Ceviche, Mango-Ginger, 207

Siegel, Dave, 96
signaling molecules, 21–22
six week plan and recipes, 173–236
  week 1: leafy greens, 175–91
  week 2: rainbows, 191–201
  week 3: seafood, 202–12
  week 4: nuts, seeds, and legumes, 213–22
  week 5: good microbiome bugs, 222–31
  week 6: growing your food roots, 232–34
skillets, 156, 159
skin conductance, 86
sleep, foods improving quality of, 14, 44, 74, 92, 104
sleep issues, 9, 12, 16, 71
slow cookers, 159, 168
Small, Scott A., 110
SMART goals, 149–50, 152, 174, 176
SMILES study, 29–31, 59, 134–35
smoked salmon, 183, 195, 202, 204
smoking, 71
Smoothie, Chocolate Peanut Butter Cup, 225
Smoothie, Kefir Berry, 225–26
smoothies
  berries and fruits in, 143–44, 176, 224, 225–26
  formulas for, 224
  frozen foods and, 166–67, 226
  kefir in, 92, 132, 143–44, 176, 224, 225–26, 231
  leafy greens in, 5, 102, 143–44, 150, 176, 225, 226
  nuts and seeds in, 106, 176, 213, 221, 224, 225–26
  vegetables in, 124
  yogurt in, 223
snacks, 5, 106, 108, 170, 213, 214, 221
Soba Dashi with Poached Egg, 209–10

socially evaluated cold pressor task, 86–87

sodium, 24

soil health, 109

soups. *See also* Caldo Verde; Coconut-Ginger Lentil Soup; Miso Butternut Squash Soup

herbs and spices in, 162, 163, 164, 217

leafy greens and, 102, 124, 176, 178, 189, 216–17

nuts, beans, and seeds in, 106, 124, 213, 214, 226–27

rainbows in, 216–17

sour cream, 185, 187, 208

sourdough and sourdough bread, 110, 134, 195, 230

spices, 164–65

spinach, 102, 167

in recipes, 179, 186, 189, 190–91, 197–98, 199, 200–201, 216–17

six week plan and, 175, 176, 178

vitamins and minerals in, 14, 35, 36, 40

sprouts, 98–99, 176, 195

SSRIs, 10, 61, 70

STAR*D, 10

statins, 69–70

steak, 48

steel-cut oatmeal, 161

stews, 104, 106, 124, 163, 164

stir-fries, 102, 104, 166, 167, 169, 177, 178, 194

storage containers, 156, 159

strawberries, 47, 166, 192

stress, 67, 71, 83–84, 89, 111–12

stress hormones, 9, 62, 83, 86, 89

stress response and bacteria, 84–88, 92, 94

strokes, 25, 131–32

sugar, 23, 24, 71, 101, 108, 112, 130–31, 223

sukuma wiki, 96

sulforaphane, 121

sunflower butter, 220

sunflower seeds, 42, 183, 187, 188, 195, 196, 221

SUN Navarra study, 26, 27

superfoods, 15, 97–99, 113, 128, 166

supertasters, 123–24

supplements, 33, 46, 90–91, 94, 120–22

Susan, 6–7, 77–78, 85, 92–93, 117–19, 143, 177

sushi, 100, 212

Swadoosh, Jessica, 96

sweet potatoes, 14, 43, 191–92, 193

Sweet Potatoes, Crispy Pan-Seared, 196–97

Swiss chard, 40, 99, 179, 186, 189, 190–91

synapses, 38, 44, 46–47, 49, 61, 62, 63, 70, 74

takeout meals, 169

tarragon, 163

teas, 98–99, 132, 133

tempeh, 93

thiamine. *See* vitamin B1 (thiamine)

thinking, clarity of, 34, 35, 111

thyme, 163, 200, 204, 218

thyroid gland and thyroid function, 14, 41, 42, 103

tomatoes

basil and, 162

lycopene in, 192

rainbow food category and, 103, 104, 193

in recipes, 179, 182, 184–85, 200–201, 208–9, 216–17, 218

tongs, 156, 157

toolkit, kitchen, 156, 157–59, 170

toxins

BDNF and, 62, 63

fiber and elimination of, 93
inflammatory system and, 67, 71
in seafood, 105, 125, 203
in vitamin supplements, 121
trans fats (trans-unsaturated fatty
acids), 23, 24, 62, 71, 72, 166
trout, 42
Truffles, Chocolate Brain, 220
Trust Me, I'm a Doctor (TV show),
91–92
tryptophan, 45
tuna, 37, 41, 183, 212
turkey, ground, 15, 48, 200–201
Turkey Zucchini Skillet Lasagna,
200–201
turmeric, 165, 179, 216–17

ulcerative colitis, 66

vaccenic acid, 51
vagus nerve, 89
Val66Met polymorphism, 62–64
vegan diets, 46, 101, 118, 126,
127–28, 185, 215
vegetable oils, 23–24, 26
vegetable peelers, 156, 157
vegetables. *See also* leafy greens;
rainbows; *specific vegetables*
added to brown rice, 132
nutrients in, 40, 93, 94
frozen, 193
ghee and, 166
herbs added to, 162
inflammation and lack of, 71, 72
Mediterranean diet and, 25, 32, 75
in recipes, 124, 194
takeout meals and, 169
vegetarian diets, 36, 46, 48, 126,
127–28, 159, 217
vinegar, 36, 186, 188, 197–98, 199,
209–10, 227–29
vision, 43

vitamin A, 14, 17, 43, 44, 98, 102,
107, 176, 121, 191–92
vitamin B1 (thiamine), 14, 17,
42–44, 82, 160, 227
vitamin B6, 14, 17, 44–45, 128, 164,
212, 221
vitamin B9. *See* folate
vitamin B12 (cobalamin), 14–15,
17, 22, 45–46, 105–107, 126,
128, 202, 205, 212, 227
vitamin C, 15, 17, 47–48, 98, 102,
164, 176, 178
vitamin D, 121, 128
vitamin E, 104, 107
vitamin K, 99, 176
vitamins and minerals. *See also*
specific vitamins and minerals
brain function and health and,
5–6, 12, 22, 33, 65
in clams, 210
in dark chocolate, 36, 74, 111, 220
food categories and, 98, 99, 112
in grass-fed animal products, 107,
166
in leafy greens/leaves, 96, 99,
176, 177
in nuts, beans, and seeds, 105–6,
161
in spices, 164
in supplements, 33, 46, 120–22
in whole grains, 161
vitamin synthesis, 81, 82, 83

walnuts, 64, 75–76, 99, 106, 176,
183, 187, 213, 221
watercress, 102, 124, 175, 176, 178
weight gain or loss, 51, 122–23
Western diet, 24, 26, 60, 72, 91,
222
wheat, 133, 134
white beans, 14, 226
white blood cells, 65

Whitehall II study, 131
white matter of the brain, 5–6
whole-foods-based diets, 72, 75, 113
  whole grains, 14, 20, 25, 32, 72,
    93, 134, 135, 160–61. *See also
    specific grains*
wild rice, 160

yeast, nutritional, 185, 187
yogurt
  for carb craving, 132
  good microbiome bugs and, 92,
    93, 108, 110, 222, 231
  lactose intolerance and, 130
  nutrients in, 108, 109
  in recipes, 185, 187, 205, 208–9,
    217, 223
  sweeteners for, 104, 132, 223

zeaxanthin, 43
zinc
  BDNF production and, 65
  brain health and, 22
  in dark chocolate, 111
  deficiency in, 24, 98
  inflammation and, 76
  as key nutrient, 15, 17, 48–49
  in meat, eggs, and dairy category,
    109, 128
  nutritional psychiatry and, 3–4
  in nuts, beans, and seeds, 99, 105,
    217, 221
  in pork and sauerkraut, 227
  in seafood, 105, 202, 212
  in seaweed, 103
Zoloft, 10
zucchini, 162, 200–201, 209

ABOUT THE AUTHOR

DREW RAMSEY, MD, is a psychiatrist, author, and farmer. His work focuses on clinical excellence, nutritional interventions, and creative media. He is an assistant clinical professor of psychiatry at Columbia University College of Physicians and Surgeons and has an active clinical practice based in New York City.

He founded the Brain Food Clinic in New York City in 2011, offering treatment and consultation for depression, anxiety, and emotional wellness concerns. The clinic incorporates evidence-based nutrition and integrative psychiatry treatments with psychotherapy, coaching, and responsible medication management.

Dr. Ramsey is a frequent keynote speaker and conducts workshops nationally. His work has been featured in the *New York Times* and the *Wall Street Journal* and on the *Today* show, the BBC, and NPR, and he has given three TEDx talks on nutrition and mental health. He has published academic work in *Lancet Psychiatry*, *Comprehensive Psychiatry*, and the *Journal of World Psychiatry*. He is on the advisory board at *Men's Health* and the editorial board at *Medscape Psychiatry*.

He is the author of three prior books, most recently the IACP Award–winning cookbook *Eat Complete: The 21 Nutrients that Fuel Brain Power, Boost Weight Loss, and Transform Your Health*. The bestseller *Fifty Shades of Kale* made this superfood accessible to thousands. *The Happiness Diet: A Nutritional Prescription for a Sharp Brain, Balanced Mood, and Lean, Energized Body* explores the impact of modern diets on brain health.

Dr. Ramsey is a diplomate of the American Board of Psychiatry and Neurology. He completed his specialty training in adult psychiatry at Columbia University and the New York State Psychiatric Institute, received an MD from Indiana University School of Medicine, and is a Phi Beta Kappa graduate of Earlham College.

He splits his time between New York City and Crawford County, Indiana, where he lives with his wife and children on their organic farm and forest.

Learn more at DrewRamseyMD.com.